Philip McCallion, PhD, ACSW
Matthew Janicki, PhD
Editors

Grandparents as Carers of Children with Disabilities: Facing the Challenges

Grandparents as Carers of Children with Disabilities: Facing the Challenges has been co-published simultaneously as *Journal of Gerontological Social Work*, Volume 33, Number 3 2000

Pre-Publication
REVIEWS,
COMMENTARIES,
EVALUATIONS . . .

"**I**NTRIGUING. . . . While particularly helpful to social workers and policymakers, this volume casts a wider, uncompromising light on the truth that kinship foster care is not a soft option, but it need not be second-best for anyone."

Patricia Noonan Walsh, PhD
Professor
Centre for the Study
of Developmental Disabilities
National University of Ireland, Dublin

"**D**rs. McCallion and Janicki have edited a very important volume on grandparents raising children with disabilities. The number of custodial grandparents continues to increase with one estimate suggesting that about one in ten grandparents will raise grandchildren at some point in their lives. Due to the social conditions that precipitate grandparent care, such as HIV/AIDS, drug use, and abuse/neglect, the children in custody of grandparents may have challenging behavioral, physical, and emotional needs. This volume specifically addresses children with disabilities to highlight both the challenges for and resilience of their grandparent caregivers.

This volume will be beneficial for a variety of audiences. Since more human service professionals are working with these intergenerational families, this book will provide additional practice and program content to construct more responsive service delivery systems. In addition, researchers and academics with expertise in child welfare, aging, and disabilities will find the studies in this volume an important contribution to the literature. In addition, students can use this material to gain knowledge of critical practice, policy and research issues.

Taking as a whole, the chapters provide a good summary of both practice and policy issues for grandparent-carers. This manuscript is an important addition to the literature, and looks at those grandparents who are faced with additional challenges by raising their grandchildren who have various types of disabilities."

Nancy P. Kropf, PhD
Associate Dean
School of Social Work
University of Georgia

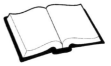

Grandparents as Carers of Children with Disabilities: Facing the Challenges

Grandparents as Carers of Children with Disabilities: Facing the Challenges has been co-published simultaneously as *Journal of Gerontological Social Work*, Volume 33, Number 3 2000.

The *Journal of Gerontological Social Work* Monographic "Separates"

Below is a list of "separates," which in serials librarianship means a special issue simultaneously published as a special journal issue or double-issue *and* as a "separate" hardbound monograph. (This is a format which we also call a "DocuSerial.")

"Separates" are published because specialized libraries or professionals may wish to purchase a specific thematic issue by itself in a format which can be separately cataloged and shelved, as opposed to purchasing the journal on an on-going basis. Faculty members may also more easily consider a "separate" for classroom adoption.

"Separates" are carefully classified separately with the major book jobbers so that the journal tie-in can be noted on new book order slips to avoid duplicate purchasing.

You may wish to visit Haworth's website at . . .

http://www.HaworthPress.com

. . . to search our online catalog for complete tables of contents of these separates and related publications.

You may also call 1-800-HAWORTH (outside US/Canada: 607-722-5857), or Fax 1-800-895-0582 (outside US/Canada: 607-771-0012), or e-mail at:

getinfo@haworthpressinc.com

Grandparents as Carers of Children with Disabilities: Facing the Challenges, edited by Philip McCallion, PhD, ACSW, and Matthew Janicki, PhD (Vol. 33, No. 3, 2000). *Here is the first comprehensive consideration of the unique needs and experiences of grandparents caring for children with developmental disabilities. The vital information found here will assist practitioners, administrators, and policymakers to include the needs of this special population in the planning and delivery of services, and it will help grandparents in this situation to better care for themselves as well as for the children in their charge.*

Latino Elders and the Twenty-First Century: Issues and Challenges for Culturally Competent Research and Practice, edited by Melvin Delgado, PhD (Vol. 30, No. 1/2, 1998). *Explores the challenges that gerontological social work will encounter as it attempts to meet the needs of the growing number of Latino elders utilizing culturally competent principles.*

Dignity and Old Age, edited by Rose Dobrof, DSW, and Harry R. Moody, PhD (Vol. 29, No. 2/3, 1998). *"Challenges us to uphold the right to age with dignity, which is embedded in the heart and soul of every man and woman." (H. James Towey, President, Commission on Aging with Dignity, Tallahassee, FL)*

Intergenerational Approaches in Aging: Implications for Education, Policy and Practice, edited by Kevin Brabazon, MPA, and Robert Disch, MA (Vol. 28, No. 1/2/3, 1997). *"Provides a wealth of concrete examples of areas in which intergenerational perspectives and knowledge are needed." (Robert C. Atchley, PhD, Director, Scribbs Gerontology Center, Miami University)*

Social Work Response to the White House Conference on Aging: From Issues to Actions, edited by Constance Corley Saltz, PhD, LCSW (Vol. 27, No. 3, 1997). *"Provides a framework for the discussion of issues relevant to social work values and practice, including productive aging, quality of life, the psychological needs of older persons, and family issues." (Jordan I. Kosberg, PhD, Professor and PhD Program Coordinator, School of Social Work, Florida International University, North Miami, FL)*

Special Aging Populations and Systems Linkages, edited by M. Joanna Mellor, DSW (Vol. 25, No. 1/2, 1996). *"An invaluable tool for anyone working with older persons with special needs." (Irene Gutheil, DSW, Associate Professor, Graduate School of Social Service, Fordham University)*

New Developments in Home Care Services for the Elderly: Innovations in Policy, Program, and Practice, edited by Lenard W. Kaye, DSW (Vol. 24, No. 3/4, 1995). *"An excellent compilation. . . .*

Especially pertinent to the functions of administrators, supervisors, and case managers in home care. . . . Highly recommended for every home care agency and a must for administrators and middle managers." (Geriatric Nursing Book Review)

Geriatric Social Work Education, edited by M. Joanna Mellor, DSW, and Renee Solomon, DSW (Vol. 18, No. 3/4, 1992). *"Serves as a foundation upon which educators and fieldwork instructors can build courses that incorporate more aging content."* (SciTech Book News)

Vision and Aging: Issues in Social Work Practice, edited by Nancy D. Weber, MSW (Vol. 17, No. 3/4, 1992). *"For those involved in vision rehabilitation programs, the book provides practical information and should stimulate readers to revise their present programs of care."* (Journal of Vision Rehabilitation)

Health Care of the Aged: Needs, Policies, and Services, edited by Abraham Monk, PhD (Vol. 15, No. 3/4, 1990). *"The chapters reflect firsthand experience and are competent and informative. Readers . . . will find the book rewarding and useful. The text is timely, appropriate, and well-presented."* (Health & Social Work)

Twenty-Five Years of the Life Review: Theoretical and Practical Considerations, edited by Robert Disch, MA (Vol. 12, No. 3/4, 1989). *This practical and thought-provoking book examines the history and concept of the life review.*

Gerontological Social Work: International Perspectives, edited by Merl C. Hokenstad, Jr., PhD, and Katherine A. Kendall, PhD (Vol. 12, No. 1/2, 1988). *"Makes a very useful contribution in examining the changing role of the social work profession in serving the elderly."* (Journal of the International Federation on Ageing)

Gerontological Social Work Practice with Families: A Guide to Practice Issues and Service Delivery, edited by Rose Dobrof, DSW (Vol. 10, No. 1/2, 1987). *An in-depth examination of the importance of family relationships within the context of social work practice with the elderly.*

Ethnicity and Gerontological Social Work, edited by Rose Dobrof, DSW (Vol. 9, No. 4, 1987). *"Addresses the issues of ethnicity with great sensitivity. Most of the topics addressed here are rarely addressed in other literature."* (Dr. Milada Disman, Department of Behavioral Science, University of Toronto)

Social Work and Alzheimer's Disease, edited by Rose Dobrof, DSW (Vol. 9, No. 2, 1986). *"New and innovative social work roles with Alzheimer's victims and their families in both hospital and non-hospital settings."* (Continuing Education Update)

Gerontological Social Work Practice in the Community, edited by George S. Getzel, DSW and M. Joanna Mellor, DSW (Vol. 8, No. 3/4, 1985). *"A wealth of information for all practitioners who deal with the elderly. An excellent reference for faculty, administrators, clinicians, and graduate students in nursing and other service professions who work with the elderly."* (American Journal of Care for the Aging)

Gerontological Social Work in Home Health Care, edited by Rose Dobrof, DSW (Vol. 7, No. 4, 1984). *"A useful window onto the home health care scene in terms of current forms of service provided to the elderly and the direction of social work practice in this field today."* (PRIDE Institute Journal)

The Uses of Reminiscence: New Ways of Working with Older Adults, edited by Marc Kaminsky (Vol. 7, No. 1/2, 1984). *"Rich in ideas for anyone working with life review groups."* (Guidepost)

A Healthy Old Age: A Sourcebook for Health Promotion with Older Adults, edited by Stephanie FallCreek, MSW, and Molly K. Mettler, MSW (Vol. 6, No. 2/3, 1984). *"An outstanding text on the 'how-tos' of health promotion for elderly persons."* (Physical Therapy)

Gerontological Social Work Practice in Long-Term Care, edited by George S. Getzel, DSW, and M. Joanna Mellor, DSW (Vol. 5, No. 1/2, 1983). *"Veteran practitioners and graduate social work students will find the book insightful and a valuable prescriptive guide to the do's and don'ts of practice in their daily work."* (The Gerontologist)

Grandparents as Carers of Children with Disabilities: Facing the Challenges has been co-published simultaneously as *Journal of Gerontological Social Work*, Volume 33, Number 3 2000.

The Haworth Press, Inc., 10 Alice Street, Binghamton, NY 13904-1580 USA

Cover design by Thomas J. Mayshock Jr.

Library of Congress Cataloging-in-Publication Data

Grandparents as carers of children with disabilities: facing the challenges/Philip McCallion, Matthew Janicki, editors
     p. cm.
    Includes bibliographical references and index.
    ISBN 0-7890-1192-1 (alk. paper)–ISBN 0-7890-1193-X (alk. paper)
    1. Hanbdicapped children–Care. 2. Grandparents as parents. 3. Caregivers. 4. Child care.
    I. McCallion, Philip. II. Janicki, Matthew P., 1943-
HV888 .G73 2000
362.4'048'0830973–dc21

00-057551

Grandparents as Carers of Children with Disabilities: Facing the Challenges

Philip McCallion, PhD, ACSW
Matthew Janicki, PhD
Editors

Grandparents as Carers of Children with Disabilities: Facing the Challenges has been co-published simultaneously as *Journal of Gerontological Social Work*, Volume 33, Number 3 2000.

The Haworth Press Inc.
New York • London • Oxford

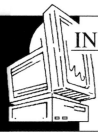

INDEXING & ABSTRACTING

Contributions to this publication are selectively indexed or abstracted in print, electronic, online, or CD-ROM version(s) of the reference tools and information services listed below. This list is current as of the copyright date of this publication. See the end of this section for additional notes.

- *Abstracts in Social Gerontology: Current Literature on Aging*

- *Academic Abstracts/CD-ROM*

- *Academic Search: data base of 2,000 selected academic serials, updated monthly: EBSCO Publishing*

- *AgeInfo CD-Rom*

- *AgeLine Database*

- *Alzheimer's Disease Education & Referral Center (ADEAR)*

- *Applied Social Sciences Index & Abstracts (ASSIA) (Online: ASSI via Data-Star) (CDRom: ASSIA Plus)*

- *Behavioral Medicine Abstracts*

- *Biosciences Information Service of Biological Abstracts (BIOSIS)*

- *Brown University Geriatric Research Application Digest "Abstracts Section"*

- *caredata CD: the social & community care database*

- *CINAHL (Cumulative Index to Nursing & Allied Health Literature), in print, also on CD-ROM from CD PLUS, EBSCO, and SilverPlatter, and online from CDP Online (formerly BRS), Data-Star, and PaperChase. (Support materials include Subject Heading List, Database Search Guide, and instructional video.)*

- *CNPIEC Reference Guide: Chinese National Directory of Foreign Periodicals*

- *Criminal Justice Abstracts*

(continued)

- *Current Contents: Clinical Medicine/Life Sciences (CC:CM/LS) (weekly Table of Contents Service), and Social Science Citation Index. Articles also searchable through Social SciSearch, ISI's online database and in ISI's Research Alert current awareness service*

- *Expanded Academic Index*

- *Family Studies Database (online and CD/ROM)*

- *Family Violence & Sexual Assault Bulletin*

- FINDEX <www.publist.com>

- *Human Resources Abstracts (HRA)*

- *IBZ International Bibliography of Periodical Literature*

- *Index to Periodical Articles Related to Law*

- *MasterFILE: updated database from EBSCO Publishing*

- *National Center for Chronic Disease Prevention & Health Promotion (NCCDPHP)*

- *National Clearinghouse for Primary Care Information (NCPCI)*

- *New Literature on Old Age*

- *Periodical Abstracts, Research I (general & basic reference indexing & abstracting data-base from University Microfilms International (UMI))*

- *Periodical Abstracts, Research II (broad coverage indexing & abstracting data-base from University Microfilms International (UMI))*

- *Psychological Abstracts (PsycINFO)*

- *Social Services Abstracts <www.csa.com>*

- *Social Science Source*

- *Social Sciences Index (from Volume 1 & continuing)*

- *Social Work Abstracts*

- *Sociological Abstracts (SA) <www.csa.com>*

(continued)

Special Bibliographic Notes related to special journal issues
(separates) and indexing/abstracting:

- indexing/abstracting services in this list will also cover material in any "separate" that is co-published simultaneously with Haworth's special thematic journal issue or DocuSerial. Indexing/abstracting usually covers material at the article/chapter level.
- monographic co-editions are intended for either non-subscribers or libraries which intend to purchase a second copy for their circulating collections.
- monographic co-editions are reported to all jobbers/wholesalers/approval plans. The source journal is listed as the "series" to assist the prevention of duplicate purchasing in the same manner utilized for books-in-series.
- to facilitate user/access services all indexing/abstracting services are encouraged to utilize the co-indexing entry note indicated at the bottom of the first page of each article/chapter/contribution.
- this is intended to assist a library user of any reference tool (whether print, electronic, online, or CD-ROM) to locate the monographic version if the library has purchased this version but not a subscription to the source journal.
- individual articles/chapters in any Haworth publication are also available through the Haworth Document Delivery Service (HDDS).

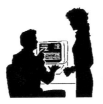

Grandparents as Carers of Children with Disabilities: Facing the Challenges

CONTENTS

ABOUT THE EDITORS

Philip McCallion, PhD, ACSW, is Associate Professor in the School of Social Welfare at the University at Albany, a Hartford Geriatric Social Work Faculty Scholar, and Associate Director of the Institute of Gerontology. Dr. McCallion's research is focused on caregiving issues, particularly the interaction of informal care with formal services, and the experiences of multicultural families. His work has addressed improving interactions between service providers in the fields of aging and developmental disabilities, developing strategies for reaching families that are not connected to service systems, demonstrating the effectiveness of empowerment-based group interventions for grandparent caregivers, and evaluation of nursing home-based, non-pharmacological interventions for persons with dementia. Many of Dr. McCallion's activities have been supported by grants and awards from the Joseph P. Kennedy, Jr. Foundation, the John A. Hartford Foundation, Reaching Up Inc., the Agency for Health Care Policy and Research, the Administration on Aging, the Alzheimer's Association, and New York State's Department of Health (Office of Mental Retardation and Developmental Disabilities, Office of Mental Health, and Office for the Aging).

Dr. McCallion has published on interventions with those who care for frail elderly people, persons with Alzheimer's disease, and persons with developmental disabilities. He is co-author of *Maintaining Communication with Persons with Dementia*. Dr. McCallion has also written on management issues for human services providers and is co-editor of *Total Quality Management in the Social Services: Theory and Practice*.

Matthew Janicki, PhD, is Research Associate Professor of Human Development and Director for Technical Assistance at the Rehabilitation Research and Training Center on Aging with Intellectual Disability at the University of Illinois at Chicago. He is the author of numerous publications on aging, dementia, rehabilitation, and intellectual disabilities. His most recent books are *Dementia, Aging, and Intellectual Disabilities* and *Community Supports for Aging Adults with Lifelong Disabilities*. He has lectured and provided training workshops around the United States and Europe. Dr. Janicki currently serves as Chair of the

United States International Council on Mental Retardation and Developmental Disabilities and as Chair of the Aging Special Interest Research Group of the International Association for the Scientific Study of Intellectual Disabilities.

Foreword

The phenomenon of grandparents becoming the primary caregivers of children in the family is not new. I remember from my childhood more than a half a century ago in Denver, Colorado three of my classmates who were being cared for by grandmothers. The mother of one was a long-term patient in the National Jewish Hospital, the tuberculosis hospital of that era, and she and her brother and her father lived for some years in the home of the grandparents, with the grandmother being *in locus* the mother. The father of another was dead, and the maternal grandmother had moved in with my classmate and her mother, who worked full-time as a secretary. Again the grandmother was the key caregiver of the grandchild. The parents of my third classmate had been killed in an automobile accident, and one set of grandparents had become the foster parents of their orphaned grandchildren.

Those experiences of my childhood I recount, because although each was tragic in its own way, they were, alas, not rare in many communities: Pneumonia and flu and tuberculosis and automobile or industrial accidents took some young parents to early graves; there were mothers and fathers who were mentally ill and hospitalized in our state mental hospitals for many years, and in some cases, for the rest of their days. And there were children living with grandparents because of the financial inability of their parents to take care of them; and there were fathers, unable to support their families, who abandoned them.

So caregiving grandparents (or "carers" in the parlance of Matthew P. Janicki and Philip McCallion, the co-editors of this volume) are not unique to this era. What is new, however, is the number of caregiving grandparents, the number of children being cared for by their grandparents, the reasons for these arrangements, and finally, the number of children with special problems included in this group. One primary reason for this increase is not the subject of this volume, but does require acknowledgement; that is, the number of

[Haworth co-indexing entry note]: "Foreword." Dobrof, Rose. Co-published simultaneously in *Journal of Gerontological Social Work* (The Haworth Press, Inc.) Vol. 33, No. 3, 2000, pp. xvii-xviii; and: *Grandparents as Carers of Children with Disabilities: Facing the Challenges* (ed: Philip McCallion and Matthew Janicki) The Haworth Press, Inc., 2000, pp. xv-xvi. Single or multiple copies of this article are available for a fee from The Haworth Document Delivery Service [1-800-342-9678, 9:00 a.m. - 5:00 p.m. (EST). E-mail address: getinfo@haworthpressinc.com].

children whose parents are absent because of the substance abuse and/or HIV/AIDS of their parents.

It is the increased number of grandparents who are caring for children with special needs that is the focus of this volume. It should be noted here that we are witness to the increase in the number of children with special problems being cared for in the community, as a function of the de-institionalization of such children. Thirty years ago, many of the children who are the subjects of the chapters in this volume would have been cared for in the large institutions for children with mental retardation which were to be found in every state in our nation.

One chapter in this volume provides an excellent picture of why this increase, and all of the chapters will help the readers understand the situations of these grandparents and the urgency of their need for help from agencies in *both* the aging network *and* the mental retardation/developmental disabilities network.

Social workers need to increase their knowledge about the service needs of both grandparents and grandchildren, and increase also their commitment to these grandparents who are in so many cases waging so heroic a battle on behalf of their grandchildren. We think all of the papers included in this volume will enhance and deepen our readers' understanding of the problems and stresses these grandparents experience. We hope this volume will be widely read, and will inspire members of our profession to meet the service needs of the grandparents and the children for whom they care.

A salute to Matthew P. Janicki and Philip McCallion for this volume, and for the contributions both have made, Phil in his role as a member of the faculty of the SUNY/Albany School of Social Work and Matt as a now retired state official, to the cause of people with special needs and their families. They are heroes in the struggle to bring people with mental retardation and developmental disabilities and their families to public attention, and to insure that these families receive the help they need.

Rose Dobrof, DSW

Preface

Increasingly there has been more attention paid to the status and condition of grandparents assuming responsibility for their grandchild because the child's parents are no longer able or available to provide care. Statistics show that one out of ten grandparents are assuming this responsibility; this suggests that primary childcare is rapidly becoming a normative experience of grandparenting. The reasons for this growing phenomenon of grandparent care have been well documented, as have the stresses and strains associated with care, and the rewards of such responsibilities. Grandparent primary care is found among all ethnic groups, and across all socioeconomic levels of society. Substance abuse, child neglect, imprisonment, AIDS/HIV, and death are primary among the reasons for parents no longer being able to provide care. Concern over preserving the family often causes grandparents to assume responsibility in spite of their limited financial means or own health condition. Such grandparent carers are overly concentrated in urban, often low income neighborhoods. Yet, even with so much that is known, little discussion has dwelt on the conditions and prevalence of grandparents caring for children with developmental delay or disabilities in these family situations. To address this, we have designed this special volume to highlight this particular situation and provide a forum for recent research examining these families and their unique circumstances.

The articles we have included in this special volume (and in the next issue of *JGSW*) show that grandparents caring for a child with a disability have many of the same concerns as other grandparent carers. Yet, they also show that grandparents caring for children with disabilities experience different and additional stresses and strains. From what we have observed, there is no question that specific targeting of grandparents caring for children with disabilities appears appropriate. First, the reasons for assuming care (for example, parental substance abuse and child neglect) are high risk factors for

[Haworth co-indexing entry note]: "Preface." McCallion, Philip, and Matthew P. Janicki. Co-published simultaneously in *Journal of Gerontological Social Work* (The Haworth Press, Inc.) Vol. 33, No. 3, 2000, pp. xix-xxi; and: *Grandparents as Carers of Children with Disabilities: Facing the Challenges* (ed: Philip McCallion and Matthew Janicki) The Haworth Press, Inc., 2000, pp. xvii-xix. Single or multiple copies of this article are available for a fee from The Haworth Document Delivery Service [1-800-342-9678, 9:00 a.m. - 5:00 p.m. (EST). E-mail address: getinfo@haworthpressinc.com].

xvii

causing and aggravating the problems and disabilities found among the children. Second, in the absence of understanding of the extent of such caregiving, local social services and disability agencies are seemingly unprepared to provide needed services. Third, many of these grandparents suffer from "service-neglect," which shows up in the many unmet needs they have (and that their grandchildren have).

The studies reported by our authors document many unmet needs for both the grandparent and the grandchild. Not only do grandparents report needs for more services for the children being cared for, but they also appear to be not addressing significant health and mental health needs of their own. These impressions are consistent with the overall grandparenting literature. What appears unique is the variety of services and the specialized services that the children with disabilities need. There is clearly a need for better understanding and better coordination between the foster care and developmental disabilities service systems, the schools, as well as the health and aging service systems. A concern about consistency of services also emerges. It is not enough to be connected with service systems. Particularly in the health arena, changes in coverages and eligibility requirements are reported to threaten consistency of care for very vulnerable young children with disabilities, and at times require intensive agency support for grandparents to successfully negotiate. For the grandparents themselves, the difficulties they experience in obtaining services add to their stress, and the lack of attention to their own needs increase risks that their care will be interrupted. One recommendation that emerges is that we need more systematic efforts to be undertaken that determine the prevalence of such children in grandparenting care situations. We need to know who, where, and when. A second recommendation is that we need additional demonstration projects that model greater coordination of services and outreach by aging, developmental disabilities, foster care, health and educational services providers. Such demonstrations should include cross training of agency staff and efforts to develop single points of entry and to reduce service access barriers and stigma.

Two other considerations deserve particular attention. One is the high level of depressive symptoms reported in a number of the studies. This deserves further investigation. The studies reported here utilized self-report measures of depression. Clearly, further studies utilizing clinical assessment measures are needed to confirm these findings. Work is also needed on developing interventions that target the grandparents' symptoms. Secondly, the process of assuming care should be examined. Neikrug (this volume) and Heller (next issue of *JGSW*) examine the relationship between grandparents and grandchildren with disabilities, independent of primary caregiving. They suggest the possibility that the caring relationship between grandparent and children with disabilities may already be different prior to the assumption of primary care. In addition, Force (next issue of *JGSW*) leads us to believe that the nature of assuming care may be significantly different among grandparents of children with early childhood disabilities (when compared to grandparents who assume care for a child free of any noticeable disability). An exploration of both the existence and meaning of differences in the way in which care is assumed for this population would be helpful to practitioners and may help further understanding of all grandparent care situations.

Philip McCallion, PhD, ACSW
Matthew P. Janicki, PhD
University at Albany

NOTE

Partial support for the development of this special volume was provided by grants from the Joseph P. Kennedy, Jr., Foundation and the National Institute on Rehabilitation and Disability Research, as well as a Geriatric Social Work Faculty Award from the John A. Hartford Foundation.

Latino Grandparents Rearing Grandchildren with Special Needs: Effects on Depressive Symptomatology

Denise Burnette, PhD, ACSW

SUMMARY. This paper examines correlates of self-reported depressive symptoms among a sample of 74 urban Latino grandparent caregivers. Nearly half of grandparents in the study scored above the clinical threshold score on the Geriatric Depression Scale, and those rearing grandchildren with special needs reported significantly more depressive symptoms than those who were not. This differential level of depressive symptoms held even with the effects of other known risk and protective factors held constant. *[Article copies available for a fee from The Haworth Document Delivery Service: 1-800-342-9678. E-mail address: <getinfo@haworthpressinc.com> Website: <http://www.HaworthPress.com>]*

KEYWORDS. Caregiving grandparents and depression, Latino grandparents, special needs grandchildren, unmet service needs

---

Denise Burnette is Associate Professor, Columbia University School of Social Work, 622 West 113th Street, New York, NY 10025 (E-mail: jdb5@columbia.edu).

The author gratefully acknowledges the contributions of Amilda Burgos, Denise Colón-Greenaway, Patricia Hernández-Kenis, Elizabeth Molina, José Ortiz, and José Tolentino.

This research was funded by the Andrus Foundation of the American Association of Retired Persons.

[Haworth co-indexing entry note]: "Latino Grandparents Rearing Grandchildren with Special Needs: Effects on Depressive Symptomatology." Burnette, Denise. Co-published simultaneously in *Journal of Gerontological Social Work* (The Haworth Press, Inc.) Vol. 33, No. 3, 2000, pp. 1-16; and: *Grandparents as Carers of Children with Disabilities: Facing the Challenges* (ed: Philip McCallion and Matthew Janicki) The Haworth Press, Inc., 2000, pp. 1-16. Single or multiple copies of this article are available for a fee from The Haworth Document Delivery Service [1-800-342-9678, 9:00 a.m. - 5:00 p.m. (EST). E-mail address: getinfo@haworthpressinc.com].

DEPRESSIVE SYMPTOMATOLOGY AMONG LATINO GRANDPARENTS REARING GRANDCHILDREN WITH SPECIAL NEEDS

Two newly emerging caregiver populations, grandparents who are rearing grandchildren and aging parents who are life-long caregivers of adult children with chronic developmental and emotional disabilities, have heightened attention to the expanding roles of older adults as family caregivers. A large body of literature on filial and spousal caregiving has documented substantial negative effects of caregiving on caregivers' well-being across multiple domains of well-being, including financial strain and physical, social, and mental health (for comprehensive reviews, see Brody, 1990; Horowitz, 1985; Schulz, Visintainer, & Williamson, 1990). Recent studies suggest that these negative sequelae of caregiving also hold for grandparents (Burnette, in press; Burton, 1992) and aging parents (Greenberg, Seltzer, & Greenley, 1993; Pruchno, Patrick, & Burant, 1996). Indeed, grandparents may be most adversely affected as they tend to bring histories of hardship to the role (Strawbridge, Wallhagen, Shema, & Kaplan, 1997) and their young charges are often beset with developmental, behavioral, and emotional difficulties associated with the circumstances leading up to grandparent care (Hayslip, Shore, Henderson, & Lambert, 1998; Pruchno, 1999).

The estimated lifetime incidence of surrogate parenting for American grandparents is 10.9%, and care extends beyond 3 years for 56% of grandparents (Fuller-Thomson, Minkler, & Driver, 1997). At present, 2.4 million or 7% of families with children under age 18 are maintained by grandparents, up 19% since 1990 (Lugaila, 1998). Ethnic minority grandmothers in families affected by social and environmental stressors in urban areas are disproportionately represented in this population–77% of custodial grandparents are women; African American grandparents are 3 times and Latinos almost twice as likely as their non-Latino white counterparts to be in a custodial role (Fuller-Thomson, Minkler, & Driver, 1997); and, 75% of children in grandparent care live in standard metropolitan areas, up from 59% just ten years ago (Harden, Clark, & Maguire, 1997).

In her review of social influences on depression in later life, George (1992) emphasizes the strong link between demographic variables which denote social location and resources and risk of depression. At all ages, women, urban residents, and persons of low socioeconomic status are at greater risk of depression than men, rural residents, and persons who have adequate economic resources. George also notes that stressful life events are strongly associated with increased risk of depression whereas social support is one of the most potent protective factors. With these role-related, socially located, and situational risk factors in mind, this paper will examine self-reported depressive symptoms among a purposive sample of 74 predominantly Carribean Latino custodial grandparents in New York City. Specifically, it aims to assess the impact of rearing grandchildren who have special developmental, emotional, and/or behavioral problems on depressive symptoms, over and above these known risk and protective factors.

LITERATURE REVIEW

Consistent with findings on other family caregiver groups (Brody, 1985; Hoyert & Selzer, 1992; Kramer, 1997), custodial grandparents report positive as well as negative consequences of caregiving. Virtually all studies report a deep sense of devotion, satisfaction, and pride with their grandchildren's presence, achievements, and growth. Mental health benefits include gratification, feeling useful, improved relations with some family members, and a sense of mastery and pride in meeting role demands (Pruchno, 1999). Burton (1992) and Minkler and Roe (1993) also found that some grandparents, motivated by a desire to improve and ensure their continued ability to provide care, reported improved health behaviors such as increased exercise, healthier diet, and decreased smoking and alcohol use. Despite these benefits, however, the net consequences of this unexpected, off-time role in middle and late life appear to be negative.

Research on mental health of grandparent caregivers is quite limited and most focuses on depression, a potentially debilitating condition which may diminish caregivers' quality of life and their role performance. Based on a nationally representative sample from the 1992-1994 National Survey of Families and Households, Minkler, Fuller-Thomson, Miller, and Driver (1997) estimate a 25% prevalence of significant depressive symptoms among grandparent caregivers (compared to 15% of non-caregiver peers), as assessed by the Center for Epidemiological Studies-Depression scale. Even with the effects of depression scores from five years earlier and sociodemographic variables known to affect depressive symptoms controlled, caring for a grandchild was associated with higher levels of depression in their multivariate prospective analysis.

Local studies suggest the prevalence of mental health problems may be even higher among urban, ethnic minority grandparents. In a study of 71 African American grandmothers who were rearing grandchildren in crack-affected families in Oakland, California, Minkler and Roe (1993) found that caregiving represented a major disruption in actual and anticipated life activities, and 44% rated their emotional health as fair or poor (Minkler, Roe, & Price, 1992). Similarly, 86% of the 60 African American grandparent caregivers in Burton's (1992) two urban samples reported feeling depressed or anxious most of the time, 61% were smoking more than ever before in their lives, and medical problems had worsened for 36%. Other mental health problems identified in these and other studies include anxiety, social isolation, social role restriction, and loss of a sense of mastery and control (Jendrek, 1993; Kelley, 1993; Shore & Hayslip, 1994).

Research on aging parents of adults with disabilities and the few studies of grandparent caregivers that report on the grandchildren in care offer further insights into potential correlates of depression for grandparents who are rearing children with special needs. Personal characteristics of the caregiver and recipient and the quality of their relationship affect mental health (Pruchno, Patrick, & Burant, 1996), for example, while features of the informal and formal support systems appear to mediate the association between perceptions and experiences of stress and well-being (Pearlin et al., 1990). Salient caregiver characteristics include age, marital status, socioeconomic status, and physical health (Greenberg et al., 1993; Seltzer & Krauss, 1980).

Grandparent-headed families tend to be poorer than those of filial or spousal caregivers (Strawbridge, Wallhagen, Shema, & Kaplan, 1997), and economic risks are greatest for the 46% of grandparent caregivers who are unmarried. The costs of rearing children with special needs is likely to exacerbate this strain. Several studies report that poor families are more likely to seek out-of-home placement for a family member with a developmental disability as a result of economic hardship (see Sherman & Cocozza, 1984). Physical health, which is especially salient to care of young children, has emerged as one of the strongest predictors of grandparent caregivers' well-being (Pruchno & Resch, 1989). Health-related concerns generally increase with advancing age, suggesting higher levels of distress among older grandparents. On the other hand, the caregiver role seems to represent a greater disruption in the life course of younger grandparents, and many pass the responsibility up the generational ladder, when possible (Burton & Bengston, 1985).

Research on the impact of child characteristics on the well-being of older adult caregivers, especially grandparents, is sparse. For adult children with disabilities, diagnosis, level of disability, physical health, and functional level are important (Greenberg et al., 1993). These characteristics also likely obtain for grandchildren, along with gender and age. Children usually enter grandparent care under adverse circumstances that include parental substance abuse, physical illness (including HIV/AIDS), incarceration, or mental illness. Many bring histories of prenatal or early childhood maltreatment and trauma associated with the literal or figurative loss of one or both parents. Behavioral, emotional, developmental, and academic problems are thus not unusual.

More than half of respondents reporting on a target grandchild between the ages of 6 and 11 in Pruchno's (1999) national study of African American and white grandmother caregivers in 'skipped-generation' families identified the following problems with their grandchildren: sudden changes in mood or feelings, nervous or high-strung, argumentative, trouble concentrating or paying attention, impulsive, hyperactive, stubborn, demands a lot of attention, and disobedient at home. A study by Hayslip et al. (1998) shows the negative impact of such problems. They found that grandparents rearing grandchildren with high levels of neurological, physical, emotional, or behavioral problems, who were more likely to be boys, exhibited higher levels of personal distress, lower role satisfaction and role meaning, and more deteriorated grandparent-grandchild relation-ships than did non-caregiver grandparents or those rearing children with few or no such problems.

To summarize, a rapidly growing number of grandparents are assuming primary care and responsibility for their grandchildren due to parental unwillingness or incapacity to fulfill this role. Many of these children have behavioral, emotional, and developmental needs associated with the difficult life circumstances that necessitated placement with their grandparents. In addition to the characteristics of grandparents and grandchildren and the stressors and supports that characterize the caregiving context, these special needs are expected to influence grandparents' mental health.

METHODS

Sampling. The purposive sample consisted of 74 self-identified Latinos age 50 or over who had primary or sole responsibility for at least one related child age 18 or under. The lower age limit of 50 was set to permit a focus on middle-aged and older grandparents. Nationally, only about one third (35%) of Latino children who reside with relatives are with grandparents (Harden, Clark, & Maguire, 1997). In this study, 93% of participants were grandparents, 5% were great-grandparents, and 2% were other relatives. Responsibility for a child was defined as the primary provider of daily care and in charge of decisions about the child's welfare.

Participants were recruited through neighborhood outreach and health and social service agencies serving high proportions of Latino children, elders, and families. Key service providers and community leaders were pivotal to promoting the study and identifying potential respondents. Interviewers screened referrals by telephone to ensure that each met inclusion criteria, then they scheduled an interview at a time and place convenient for the grandparent. Eighty-eight percent of interviews were conducted in Spanish, and nearly all took place in the grandparents' homes.

Data Collection. A professional Latina translator initially translated the data collection instrument from English to Spanish. One of the interviewers, who had also worked as a translator and had extensive experience with low-income, Latino elders, then reviewed each item carefully. This procedure offers a viable alternative to back translation, which often fails to assure use of correct colloquial words, symbolic meaning, and word structure with low-income, racial/ethnic populations (Zambrana, 1991). Several questions were reworded to improve colloquial relevance, and no problems with language were noted in three pretest interviews.

Six bilingual, bicultural interviewers who had experience working with older Latinos in the community completed a full-day training session on administration of the instrument, interviewing techniques, and technical aspects of the study protocol (Fowler & Mangione, 1990). The session included didactic training and experiential role-playing, with inter-rater agreement on randomly selected items from role-play interviews exceeding .85. Interviewers were matched to participants on language and in most cases on gender and nationality. Grandparents received $20.00 and a packet of information on local resources for grandparent caregivers for a single face-to-face interview which lasted about two hours.

Analytic Strategy. Univariate statistics were used to describe the sample and examine the distributions of variables of interest. Correlational methods were then used to construct composite measures of interrelated items, and bivariate associations among independent variables and scores on the Geriatric Depression Scale were examined with t-tests and Pearson's product-moment correlation coefficients. Using ordinary least squares procedures, these scores were then regressed on 7 independent variables selected from the literature and bivariate tests. Entered simultaneously, at least 10 cases are needed for each independent variable in the model (Concato, Feinstein, & Holford, 1993). Tolerance values ranged from .82-.96 for independent variables, indicating no problems with multicollinearity. Four cases were dropped due to missing data. With 7 variables in the equation, a medium to large effect size of .25 expected and a .10 probability level (due to the relatively small sample), a sample size of 70 yields statistical tests with power of .91 (Borenstein & Cohen, 1988).

Measures

Dependent Variable. Depressive symptoms were assessed by the 15-item short version of the Geriatric Depression Scale (GDS) (Sheikh & Yesavage, 1986). The scale's yes/no response format for symptom endorsement is appropriate for persons with low education and it has been validated for Spanish-speaking populations (Taussig, 1989). Indicators of depression are assigned 1 point each, then summed (0-5 = normal; 6-10 = mild depression; and 11-15 = moderate to severe depression). The absence of neurovegetative and somatic symptoms of depression on the GDS may reduce its sensitivity with Latinos, for whom somatization is often integral to the presentation of depressive illness. Baker et al. (1993) found that lowering the recommended threshold from 6 to 4 in a sample of 41 Mexican American elders improved the instrument's sensitivity from 49% to 75% (specificity was not assessed since all had affective disorders). The present study uses a Spanish-language version of the GDS (Izal & Montorio, 1993) and presents results for both criterion points.

Independent Variables. In addition to background characteristics of grandparents, health status, life stress, informal and formal support, and special needs of children in care were assessed. *Self-rated health status* was measured as excellent = 1; good = 2; fair = 3; poor = 4. A composite score of *stressful life events* was created by summing the occurrence of 11 stressors over the past year (yes = 1): death of (1) spouse, (2) close family member, (3) close friend; change in (4) marital, (5) health, (6) financial status, (7) residence, (8) household composition; (9) member of household ill; (10) self or spouse retired; and (11) family discord. Six indicators were summed to create a measure of *informal support* (yes = 1): other adult(s) present in household; visits with friends and relatives 4 or more times per week; has a confidant; help is available with child rearing; confident this help could continue indefinitely; and, number of extra-familial supports, e.g., support group, church, or senior center used regularly. *Unmet need* was examined rather than service use because all but one grandparent had used at least one service. Grandparents were presented a list of 16 health and social services for older adults, children, and families, then asked (a) whether they had used the service during the previous year and (b) whether they currently needed the service. Unmet need was calculated for each service (not used but needed = 1), and these scores were summed.

Special needs of grandchildren were determined by asking grandparents to identify up to two of the following conditions for each child in their care: social/emotional problems that cause the child distress in his or her daily life (e.g., withdrawn, unable to establish/maintain friendships, hypersensitivity, crying spells) (42%), learning disability (16%), hyperactivity (14%), chronic physical illness (14%), HIV/AIDS (1%), developmental disability or mental retardation (DD/MR) (14%), prenatal exposure or current drug or alcohol problems (5%). This measure was treated as dichotomous as 61% of families had at least one child with special needs. Age, gender, length of time in grandparent care, and legal status of the relationship were also determined for each child.

RESULTS

The mean age of grandparents in the study was 63, almost all (93%) were women, about one in five (22%) were married, and reflecting the Latino population in New York City, most were from Puerto Rico (60%) or the Dominican Republic (28%). They had lived in the United States on average 35 years, but language acculturation remained low–only 1 in 5 reported spoken English proficiency. Level of educational attainment and income were also very low. Only 27% had completed high school and with income adjusted for household size and using February, 1996 poverty estimates (U.S. Bureau of the Census, 1995), 81% of households had poverty level incomes. Demographic characteristics of grandparents who were rearing children with special needs did not differ significantly from those who were not.

On average, grandparents were rearing two grandchildren. Of the 150 children in the 74 families, 53% were boys and ages ranged from 4 months to 18 years ($M = 9.8$, $SD = 4.4$). Half had entered grandparent care at or within one year of birth. Relevant to the special needs of the children, nearly all grandparents had assumed the role as a result of parental child maltreatment (neglect or physical, emotional, and/or sexual abuse) combined with drug or alcohol problems (55%); incarceration (18%); HIV/AIDS infection (16%); other physical illness (12%); or mental illness (12%). About one quarter of the grandchildren's parents (24% of mothers and 23% of fathers) maintained regular contact with their children. The demographic characteristics of the grandchildren were not associated with grandparents' level of depression, nor were any of these characteristics associated with having special needs.

Table 1 presents bivariate comparisons of grandparents who are rearing special needs children and those who are not in terms of stressful life events and informal supports. The two groups did not differ significantly on either composite measure. A change in financial status and the death of a close family member, followed closely by change in health status and family discord were main sources of stress for grandparents during the preceding year. The latter two stressors were significantly greater for grandparents who were rearing children with special needs.

With respect to informal supports, grandparents were generally socially connected. Most reported having a confidant and frequent visits with family and friends, and four out of five had some help available with child rearing. Importantly, though, only about half of all grandparents expressed confidence in the ongoing reliability of this help–about the same proportion who had no other adults present in the household. Neither individual items nor the composite measure of informal support differed for grandparents rearing special needs children and those who were not.

Table 2 compares levels of unmet needs for commonly used health and social services for grandparents who are rearing special needs children and those who are not. With the exception of parent education and training skills and nutrition support for grandchildren, the former group had more unmet need for each service, and a significantly higher level of unmet service need

TABLE 1. Stressors and Social Supports by Grandchildren's Special Needs Status

	Child with Special Needs n = 45 (60.8%)	No Child With Special Needs n = 29 (39.2%)	Total n = 74 100%	
Stressful Life Events (%)				
Death of a spouse	2.3	6.9	4.2	
Death of close family member	37.2	48.3	41.7	
Change in marital status	4.7	6.9	5.6	
Death of a close friend	23.3	10.3	18.1	
Member of household ill	16.7	31.0	22.5	
Change in health status	44.2	24.1	36.1	p < .10
Self/spouse retire from work	19.0	31.0	23.9	
Change in financial status	40.5	44.8	42.3	
Change in where you live	12.2	3.4	8.6	
Change in household composition	19.0	13.8	16.9	
Family discord or troubles	44.2	20.7	34.7	p < .05
Informal Support				
Other adult in household	55.6	51.7	54.1	
Contact with family and friends 4 + times per week	73.3	86.2	78.4	
Confidant (%Yes)	91.1	86.2	89.2	
Has help available	80.0	89.7	83.6	
Help is reliable	53.3	51.7	52.7	
Community supports *M* (SD)	1.6 (.97)	1.5 (.78)	1.6 (.89)	

overall (t = -1.9, df = 70, p < .10). This differential well-being is also reflected in Geriatric Depression Scale scores, which ranged from 0-15 (*M* = 6, *SD* = 4) (Table 3). Using a clinical threshold of 6, 38% of grandparents were at least mildly depressed. Using the recommended cutoff score of 4 for Latinos increased this figure to 47%. Grandparents who were rearing special needs children were worse off on three quarters of GDS items and the overall scale score (t = -2.6, df = 71, p < .01).

The regression model explained 46% of the variance in GDS scores (*F* (7, 63) = 12.2, *p* < .0001) (Table 4). All variables except poverty status and number of unmet service needs made a significant contribution to the explained variance in GDS scores. Being younger and having lower levels of informal support and self-rated health were independently associated with higher GDS scores, as were higher levels of life stress and rearing children with special needs.

TABLE 2. Unmet Service Needs by Grandchildren's Special Needs Status

	Child with Special Needs n = 45 (60.8%)	No Child With Special Needs n = 29 (39.2%)	Total n = 74 100%	
Child Special Health Need	6.8%	0	4.1	
Special Education/Tutoring	17.9	5.7	12.2	
Counseling for Grandchild	9.1	6.7	8.1	
Legal Assistance	35.9	14.3	25.7	p < .10
Counseling for Grandparent	17.9	6.7	12.2	
Marital/Family Counseling	15.9	10.0	13.5	
Grandparent Support Group	43.2	33.3	39.2	
Respite Child Care Services	36.4	26.7	32.4	
Parent Education/Parent Skills Training	25.0	46.7	33.8	p < .10
Foster Care Services	9.1	0	5.4	
Nutrition (e.g., school lunch, WIC, food stamps)	9.1	23.3	14.9	p < .10
Homemaker Services	27.3	20.0	24.3	
Toll Free Hotline	54.5	36.7	47.3	p < .10
Drug/AIDS Education	22.7	16.7	20.0	

Note: Fisher's Exact Test (2-tailed) was used to determine significance level

DISCUSSION AND CONCLUSIONS

Drawing on studies of the family caregiver stress process of older adults and aging parents of adult children with disabilities, this study has explored the impact of rearing grandchildren with special needs on the mental health of Latino grandparent caregivers. Specifically, it examined the effects of rearing children with developmental, behavioral, or emotional problems on self-reported depressive symptoms after controlling for several established risk and protective factors, i.e., background characteristics, health status, life stress, and informal and formal supports.

The findings indicate that factors which result in mental health difficulties for other family caregiver populations also hold for grandparents and that rearing children who have special needs appears to pose added risks. As

TABLE 3. Descriptive Statistics of Major Study Variables by Grandchildren's Special Needs Status

	Child with Special Needs	No Child With Special Needs	Total	
	n = 45 (60.8%)	n = 29 (39.2%)	n = 74 100%	
GDS Items (yes = 1) (α = .88)				
Satisfied with life[a]	58.1	80.0	67.1	p < .05
Dropped activities and interests	65.1	63.3	64.4	
Feel life is empty	51.2	30.0	42.5	p < .10
Often get bored	53.5	20.0	39.7	p < .01
Good spirits most of the time[b]	65.1	83.3	72.6	p < .10
Afraid something bad will happen	41.9	23.3	34.2	p < .10
Feel happy most of the time[c]	67.4	73.3	69.9	
Often feel helpless	41.9	23.3	34.2	p<.10
Prefer to stay at home	55.8	56.7	56.2	
More memory problems than most	51.2	26.7	41.1	p < .05
Wonderful to be alive now[d]	81.4	86.7	83.6	
Feel pretty worthless	30.2	10.0	21.9	p < .05
Feel full of energy[e]	51.2	83.3	64.4	p < .01
Feel that your situation is hopeless	41.9	13.3	30.1	p < .01
Think most others are better off	55.8	33.3	46.6	p < .05

[a-e]These items recoded before calculating composite score
Note: Fisher's Exact Test (2-tailed) was used to determine significance level

Variable	Range	M (SD)	M (SD)	M SD
GDS	1-15	6.5 (4.5)	4.0 (3.4)	5.6 (4.3) p < .01
Self-rated health	1-4	2.8 (.83)	2.7 (.92)	2.8 (.87)
Life stressors	1-8	2.4 (1.8)	2.2 (1.6)	2.3 (1.7)
Informal support	1-8	5.1 (1.5)	5.1 (1.3)	5.1 (1.4)
Unmet service need	0-11	3.3 (2.7)	2.7 (2.0)	3.0 (2.5) p < .10

T-tests used to test for group differences

George (1992) suggests, characteristics that indicate location and resources in the social structure, i.e., race/ethnicity, class, gender, and age are operative. The 81% poverty rate for this sample of older urban Latina women is almost four times that of grandparent caregivers nationwide (23%) (Fuller-Thomson et al., 1997). Nearly uniform poverty in the sample probably accounts for its lack of significance in the multivariate analysis. Similarly, high rates of service use and persistent unmet need (on average respondents used 6 services in the prior year, yet 75% still reported unmet needs) (see Burnette,

TABLE 4. OLS Regression of Major Independent Variables on Depression (N = 70)

Variable	Beta	SE	p-value
Age	−.17	.06	.07
Poverty (yes = 1)	−.09	.94	NS
Self-Rated Health	.30	.45	.001
Life Stressors	.33	.22	.001
Informal Support	−.30	.28	.003
Unmet Service Needs (yes = 1)	.06	.16	NS
Child with Special Needs (yes = 1)	.22	.77	.02

Adjusted R^2 = .46 (SE = 3.1)
F = 9.39 (df = 7), p < .0001

1999a) may help explain why this variable did not contribute to depressive symptoms. The directionality and strength of age, health status, life stressors, and informal supports are consistent with previous research, but findings from this study raise additional issues specific to the mental health of grandparents who are rearing children with special needs. This group did not differ from other grandparents in the study on global self-rated health or composite measures of life stress and informal supports. It is difficult to know whether this is due to methodological limitations, e.g., the relatively small sample size and the global nature of these measures, but analysis of other items suggests that these remain areas of concern and potential points for intervention (Burnette, 1999b).

Self-reported health was poor or very poor across the board, but grandparents who were rearing children with special needs were twice as likely to report a change in health status during the previous year. Depending on the type and extent of disability, caring for a child with special needs requires considerable physical strength and stamina. As grandparents age and the children in their care mature, decrements in health and functioning may make it ever more difficult to manage disruptive behaviors or rigorous care plans, thereby increasing the risk of mental health problems.

Overall, grandparents in the study were socially connected, with frequent contacts with family and friends, confidants, and community supports. However, the limited availability of help from other adults and low confidence in sustained, instrumental help with child rearing suggests that helping networks are quite tenuous. The far greater likelihood of increased family discord among grandparents who were rearing children with special needs and their reports of less social contact and available help with child rearing are also troubling for this subgroup of grandparents.

These grandparents may also have some unique service needs. As noted, the study sample was generally connected to the service delivery system and grandparents whose grandchildren had special needs reported fewer unmet parent education and nutritional support needs. Despite being tied in to these services, however, they had more unmet service needs overall and in terms of legal information and an information hot-line. The legal status of grandparents' relationship to children in their care is crucial as it determines their responsibilities and rights and their eligibility for many public supports. It is also important for permanency planning since children with special needs may require ongoing specialized supports and may be more difficult to place if a grandparent dies or discontinues care. The need for a toll-free hot-line may reflect access barriers, such as greater difficulty leaving home due to trouble securing child care, transportation, etc. It may also speak to the greater effort needed to acquire the specialized types of information these grandparents need.

Several methodological limitations restrict the interpretation and application of findings from this study. The relatively small sample size makes it possible to detect only large effects in the data and the selection strategy prohibits generalization beyond the sample. Further, the cross-sectional design prohibits the determination of directionality in associations among variables and the findings are subject to the usual biases of self-report. Care was taken to ensure the accuracy of grandparents' reporting of special needs, i.e., by asking whether conditions were professionally diagnosed, but errors may have resulted from their inability to recognize and/or their reluctance to report these conditions.

Despite these limitations, this exploratory study strongly suggests that older adults who are rearing grandchildren with special developmental, behavioral, and emotional needs are at increased risk of depression, and that certain background characteristics, life stressors, and unmet informal and formal service needs may help account for this risk. Future research using larger samples should examine the differential effects of specific types of disabilities on mental health outcomes for grandparent caregivers. The influence of other child-related characteristics should also be considered. Boys are more likely to exhibit behavioral problems, for instance, whereas girls tend to experience more depression and social difficulties. The children's age may also be important, as adolescence brings novel and in many ways more challenging circumstances for parenting children with special needs.

These grandparents are also likely to require ongoing education and support around the etiology, nature, and expected course of their conditions. Many need help in accessing and using services, and providers in aging, child welfare, and school services, for example, may require specialized training in order to assist grandparents in identifying and accessing appropriate instrumental, informational, and emotional supports. Bilingual, culturally sensitive programming and service providers should help surmount the formidable barriers that exist for non-English speaking grandparents. Finally, professional and peer counseling and community and church supports, including services such as education and support groups and respite child care, could go far towards improving custodial grandparents' mental health and in turn, ensuring the current and long-term well-being of the children in their care.

REFERENCES

Baker, F.M., Espino, D.V., Robinson, B.H., & Stewart, B. (1993). Depression among elderly African Americans and Mexican Americans. *American Journal of Psychiatry, 150* (6), 987-988.

Borenstein, M. & Cohen, J. (1988). *Statistical power analysis: A computer program.* Hillsdale, NJ: Lawrence Erlbaum Associates.

Brody, E.M. (1990). *Women in the middle: Their parent-care years.* New York: Springer.

Burnette, D. (1999a). Custodial grandparents in Latino families: Patterns of service utilization and predictors of unmet need. *Social Work, 44* (1), 22-34.

Burnette, D. (1999b). Social relationships of Latino grandparent caregivers: A role theory perspective. *The Gerontologist, 39* (1), 49-58.

Burton, L.M. (1992). Black grandparents rearing grandchildren of drug-addicted parents: Stressors, outcomes, and social service needs. *The Gerontologist, 32* (6), 744-751.

Burton, L.M. & Bengtson, V.L. (1985). Black grandmothers: Issues of timing and continuity of roles. In V.L. Bengtson & J.F. Robertson (Eds.) *Grandparenthood* (pp. 61-77). Beverly Hills, CA: Sage.

Concato, J., Feinstein, A.R., & Holford, T.R. (1993). The risk of determining risk with multi-variate models. *Annals of Internal Medicine, 118*, 201-210.

Fuller-Thomson, E., Minkler, M. & Driver, D. (1997). A profile of grandparents raising grandchildren in the United States. *The Gerontologist, 37* (3), 406-411.

George, L.K. (1992). Social factors and the onset and outcome of depression. In K.W. Schaie, J.S. House, & D.G. Blazer (eds). *Aging, health behaviors, and health outcomes* (pp. 137- 159). Hillsdale, NJ: Erlbaum Associates.

Greenberg, J.S., Seltzer, M.M., & Greenley, J.R. (1993). Aging parents of adults with disabilities: The gratifications and frustrations of later-life caregiving. *The Gerontologist, 33*, 542-550.

Harden, A.W., Clark, R. & Maguire, K. (1997). *Informal and formal kinship care.* Report for the Office of the Assistant Secretary for Planning and Evaluation (Task Order HHS-100-95-0021). Washington D.C.: U.S. Department of Health and Human Services.

Hayslip, B. Jr., Shore, R.J., Henderson, C.E., & Lambert, P.L. (1998). Custodial grandparenting and the impact of grandchildren with problems on role satisfaction and role meaning. *Journal of Gerontology, 53B* (3), S164-S173.

Horowitz, A. (1985). Family caregiving to the frail elderly. In C. Eisdorfer (ed.) *Annual Review of Gerontology and Geriatrics*, Vol. 5, New York: Springer.

Hoyert, D.L. & Seltzer, M.M. (1992). Factors related to the well-being and life activities of family caregivers. *Family Relations, 41*, 74-81.

Izal, M. & Montorio, I. (1993). Adaptation of the Geriatric Depression Scale in Spain: A preliminary study. *Clinical Gerontologist, 13* (2), 83-89.

Jendrek, M.P. (1993). Grandparents who parent their grandchildren: Effects on lifestyle. *Journal of Marriage and the Family, 55*, 609-621.

Kelley, S.J. (1993). Caregiver stress in grandparents raising grandchildren. *IMAGE: Journal of Nursing Scholarship, 25* (4), 331-337.

Kramer, B.J. (1997). Gain in the caregiving experience: Where are we? What next? *The Gerontologist, 37* (2), 218-232.

Lugaila, T. (1998). U.S. Bureau of the Census, Current Population Reports, Series P20-506, *Marital status and living arrangements: March 1997*, Washington DC: USGPO.

Minkler, M., Fuller-Thomson, E., Miller, E., & Driver, D. (1997). Depression in grandparents raising grandchildren. *Archives of Family Medicine, 6*, 445-452.

Minkler, M. & Roe, K.M. (1993). *Forgotten caregivers: Grandmothers raising children of the crack cocaine epidemic*. Newbury Park, CA: Sage.

Minkler, M., Roe, K., & Price, M. (1992). The physical and emotional health of grandmothers raising grandchildren in the crack cocaine epidemic. *The Gerontologist, 32* (6), 752-761.

Pearlin, L.I., Mullan, J.T., Semple, S.J. & Skaff, M.M. (1990). Caregiving and the stress process: An overview of concepts and their measures. *The Gerontologist, 30*, 583-594.

Pruchno, R. (1999). Raising grandchildren: The experiences of black and white grandmothers. *The Gerontologist, 39* (2), 209-221.

Pruchno, R.A., Patrick, J.H., & Burant, C.J. (1996). Mental health of aging women with children who are chronically disabled: Examination of a two-factor model. *Journal of Gerontology, 51B* (6), S284-S296.

Pruchno, R.A. & Resch, N.C. (1989). Husbands, and wives as caregivers: Antecedents of depression and burden. *The Gerontologist, 29*, 159-165.

Schulz, R., Visintainer, P., & Williamson, G.M. (1990). Psychiatric and physical morbidity effects of caregiving. *Journal of Gerontology: Psychological Sciences, 45*, P181-P191.

Seltzer, M.M. & Krauss, M.W. (1989). Aging parents with adult mentally retarded children: Family risk factors and sources of support. *American Journal of Mental Retardation, 94* (3), 303-312.

Sherman, B.R. & Cocozza, J.J. (1984). Stress in families of the developmentally disabled: A literature review of factors affecting the decision to seek out-of-home placements. *Family Relations, 33*, 95-103.

Shore, R.J., & Hayslip, B. Jr. (1994). Custodial grandparenting: Implications for children's development. In A.E. Gottfried & A.W. Gottfried (Eds.) *Redefining families: Implications for children's development* (pp. 171-218). New York: Plenum Press.

Sheikh, J.I. & Yesavage, J.A. (1986). Geriatric Depression Scale (GDS): Recent evidence and development of a shorter version. In T.L. Brink (Ed.), *Clinical gerontology: A guide to assessment and intervention* (pp. 165-173). New York: The Haworth Press, Inc.

Strawbridge, W.J., Wallhagen, M.I., Shema, S.J., & Kaplan, G.A. (1997). New burdens or more of the same? Comparing grandparent, spouse, and adult child caregivers. *Gerontologist, 37* (4), 505-510.

Taussig, I.M. (1989). Translation and validation of neuropsychological and clinical batteries for Spanish-speaking Alzheimer's Disease patients. Paper presented at International Congress of Gerontology, Acapulco.

U.S. Bureau of the Census (1995). *Money Income and Poverty Status of Families and Persons in the United States.* Washington D.C.: U.S. Department of Commerce.

Zambrana, R.E. (1991). Cross-cultural methodological strategies in the study of low income racial ethnic populations. In H. Hibbard, P.A. Nutting, & M.L. Grady (Ed.), *Primary Care Research: Theory and Methods* (pp. 221-227) USDHHS, Public Health Service, Agency for Health Care Policy and Research Pub. No. 91-0011, Rockville, MD.

The Special Needs
of Children in Kinship Care

Roy Grant

SUMMARY. Over the past decade, grandparents have increasingly been called upon to raise their children's children because of family disruption often due to parental abandonment, death, or incarceration. This can be stressful for the grandparents, who may not get the financial assistance received by traditional foster parents. This article presents data from a school-based comprehensive multi-generation program in East Harlem (New York City). It explores environmental stressors associated with children coming into kinship care, and the special developmental, behavioral and school problems they may present. The impact on the grandparent caregivers is discussed, focusing on health status and access to care. *[Article copies available for a fee from The Haworth Document Delivery Service: 1-800-342-9678. E-mail address: <getinfo@haworthpressinc. com> Website: <http://www.HaworthPress.com>]*

KEYWORDS. Kinship care, special needs, grandchildren, environmental stressors, impact of caregiving on grandparents

---

Roy Grant is affiliated with The Children's Hospital at Montefiore Medical Center, Albert Einstein College of Medicine.

Address correspondence to: Roy Grant, Director, Ready For School Program, Montefiore Medical Center, Community Pediatrics, 317 East 64th Street, New York, NY 10021 (E-mail: rgrant@montefiore.org).

The Grandparent Caregivers Program was made possible by the combined efforts of The Mount Sinai Medical Center and the Brookdale Foundation Group, New York City.

[Haworth co-indexing entry note]: "The Special Needs of Children in Kinship Care." Grant, Roy. Co-published simultaneously in *Journal of Gerontological Social Work* (The Haworth Press, Inc.) Vol. 33, No. 3, 2000, pp. 17-33; and: *Grandparents as Carers of Children with Disabilities: Facing the Challenges* (ed: Philip McCallion and Matthew Janicki) The Haworth Press, Inc., 2000, pp. 17-33. Single or multiple copies of this article are available for a fee from The Haworth Document Delivery Service [1-800-342-9678, 9:00 a.m. - 5:00 p.m. (EST). E-mail address: getinfo@haworthpressinc.com].

17

Among the changes in the structure of the nuclear family over the past decade is the enormous growth of kinship care: children being raised by extended family members, typically grandparents caring for their children's children. This family composition has increased by 76% since 1970 (from 2.2 million children to 3.9 million in 1997) (National Committee to Preserve Social Security and Medicare, 1998), a change which coincides with an overall decline from 85% to 68% of children living in a two-parent family (DHHS, 1998). Also increasing is the number of children reported as abused or neglected, up 41% from 1988 to 1997, to nearly 3.2 million children, while there was a decline in the number of licensed foster care homes (Child Welfare League of America, 1999). Infants are the fastest growing age group of children entering foster care (Carnegie Corporation of New York, 1994). The result is a greater likelihood that children removed from their parents' custody will be placed with relatives, and that these children will be very young.

Grandparents have traditionally been, and continue to be, integral to extended families and important resources for parents. However, the new kinship care of the 1990's is quite different. Grandparent caregivers often become the default parent for their grandchildren when the biological parents are unavailable. Reasons include parental death (often due to AIDS or violence), substance abuse, abandonment, and incarceration. Because these social problems are often associated with poverty, the new grandparent caregiving is increasingly a feature of family structure in low income communities.

Kinship care may be either formal or informal; that is, there may or may not be official designation of the grandparent(s) or other relative(s) as foster parents. The prevalence of informal arrangements makes it difficult to make accurate estimates. However, a strong increase since 1983 is noted in United States Census Bureau (Current Population Survey) data. There is no evidence of an increase among non-Hispanic whites, the greater incidence of kinship care arrangements being seen primarily among racial and ethnic minority groups. For example, African-American children are four to five times more likely to live with relatives in the absence of their biological parents than are white children (Harden, Clark, & Maguire, 1997). In 1997, 3.8% of white children (1.6 million) lived with their grandparents, compared with 15.6% of African-American children (1.4 million). Among Hispanics, 7.4% of children, more than 600,000, lived with grandparents in the absence of their biological parents (Fuller-Thomson, Minkler, & Driver, 1997).

United States Department of Human Services (DHHS) statistics show that half of kinship caregivers are married; however, among those that are single, 85% are women. While 95% of parents who live with their children are under 50 years of age, more than half of kinship caregivers are 50 or older. Kinship caregivers, compared with parents, are more likely to be currently unmarried, less well educated, more likely to be unemployed or otherwise out of the labor force (including retired), to be poor, and to be dependent on government programs (Harden et al., 1997).

Informal arrangements are more common than formal (kinship foster care). In four states studied by the Department of Health and Human Services (New York, California, Illinois, and Missouri), only 15.5% of children in kinship care were formally placed. Children under five years of age are more than twice as likely to be in kinship foster care than children 6-17 years. Formal placements are more common in large cities. African-American children are most likely to be in a formal placement. They are eight times more likely to be in kinship foster care than children of other race and ethnicity, in the four states studied by DHHS (Harden et al., 1997).

One out of five grandparent headed households live in a rural county or small town. In large cities, it has been estimated that 30% to 50% of grandparents are primary caregivers to their grandchildren for at least six months. One fifth of grandparent caregivers remain in that role for ten years or more (Minkler, 1997). Among the children, half are under the age of six years. One third lack health insurance (U.S. Census Bureau, 1999).

The challenges of maintaining good care for the children in kinship homes can be formidable. The child's health insurance benefits may be terminated because in many cases it had been part of a family benefit package under the biological parent(s). Foster care subsidies paid to non-family foster parents may not be provided to relatives, especially if there is not a formal court placement. School problems may lead to special education referrals, and special needs of younger children involve the grandparent in other difficult systems (preschool special education and/or the Early Intervention Program). Legal issues around guardianship, custody, child care, and health services may become overwhelming, as may economic pressures (Brookdale Center on Aging, 1999). The associated stress may be deleterious to the health of the grandparent.

There are special problems with regard to maintaining custody, or adopting, for grandparents in foster care relationships. The grandparent may have to challenge the fitness to parent of the biological parent of the child in care–typically her own daughter. Court decisions often favor reunification with the biological parent even when this is not objectively in the best interests of the child. These two issues together make grandparent caregivers especially vulnerable to losing custody of the children for whom they are the caring. This is a major source of stress and potential instability for both grandparent and child (Stanton, 1998). One study which focused on kinship care placements in the early 1990's found that, compared with non-familial foster home placements, children in kinship households were less likely to have legal permanency planning (Berrick, 1994).

The health status of grandparent caregivers has been investigated. One study, using data from the National Survey of Families and Households (1992-1994), found that custodial grandparents have a 50% higher chance of having a daily activity limitation. They report lower satisfaction with their own health and rate their health status lower than do non-custodial grandparents (Minkler, & Fuller-Thomson, 1999). In a 1998 study, 70% of Hispanic grandparent caregivers rated their own health as fair or poor (Brockway, 1998).

Another recent study explored the impact of the child in care on the grandparent caregiver. There was a relationship between special needs the child presents (neurological, physical, emotional, or behavioral) and the degree of stress the grandparent experienced. More serious developmental or behavioral problems had a deteriorating effect on the grandparent-grandchild relationship. Grandparents caring for developmentally typical children also had a higher level of stress than did grandparents who were not in a child caring role (Emick, & Hayslip, 1999).

CHILDREN IN FOSTER CARE:
DEVELOPMENTAL AND MENTAL HEALTH PROBLEMS

There is an extensive literature detailing the possible developmental, emotional-behavioral, and school problems of children in foster care. One study, using school records, compared school performance for children known to have been maltreated. Two groups were matched for age, race, sex, and year of diagnosis; they differed in that one group had been removed from their biological parents' custody and placed in foster care. The foster care children were more likely to be placed in special education eight years after the reported incident of abuse or neglect, although both groups did poorly academically (Runyan, & Gould, 1985).

This study implies that child maltreatment is likely to have a negative impact on school performance, and that this is compounded by foster care placement. Two possible mechanisms are suggested. The first is that foster care necessarily disrupts the relationship between child and parent(s). In addition, a large national study found that 30% of foster children who were in care at the end of fiscal year 1990 were in three or more different foster homes, including group shelters, during the preceding three years (National Center for Policy Analysis, 1997). Frequent changes in foster placement have been identified as a problem affecting the health and development of children in foster care (Schor, 1982).

The specific problems that bring children into foster care have also been identified as having a potential negative impact on the child. Controlling for socio-economic status and other potential confounding variables, researchers found that children who suffered abuse showed pervasive and significant academic and social-emotional problems. Problems were more severe for neglected children (Kurtz, Graudin, Woodarski, & Howing, 1993). These results were corroborated by a similar subsequent study which found that neglected or abused children did more poorly in school than did non-mal-treated matched controls, characterized by lower grades, more disciplinary referrals and suspensions, and more grade retention (Kendall, & Eckenrode, 1996). Children who experienced both neglect and abuse had the most disciplinary referrals and grade retention.

These findings are consistent with the first comprehensive study of the school performance of children in kinship care. This is to be expected because kinship care is a specific kind of foster care; the reasons that children may come into kinship care can be predicted to be the same as those which bring a child into traditional foster care. In this study, children in kinship households, compared to their peers, had higher rates of grade retention and academic problems requiring remediation and/or special education. Academic achievement was lower, and speech-language and cognitive deficits were noted (Sawyer, & Dubowitz, 1994).

In addition to developmental and academic deficits, behavior problems have frequently been noted among children in foster care. A review of the literature over a 20 year period (1974-1994) revealed that the prevalence of psychopathology among children in foster care is higher than would be expected from normative data, controlling for socio-economic status and other environmental restrictions. The trend in behavioral presentation is towards externalizing disorders, specifically disruptive behavior disorders (Pilowski, 1995). A higher prevalence of emotional and behavioral problems among children in foster care was strongly revealed in a California study, which found that children in foster care accounted for 41% of all users of mental health services despite representing less than 4% of the public insurance eligible (Medi-Cal) population. Compared to their peers, children in foster care had 10 to 20 times the rate of utilization (Halfon, Berkowitz, & Klee, 1992). Similar findings came from a subsequent study in the state of Washington, which found that mental health services were used by 25% of children in foster care compared with 3% of children on public assistance and Medicaid (Takayama, Bergman, & Connell, 1994).

CONTEXT AND METHOD:
THE TWO STUDIES

As part of a comprehensive school-based health center serving four elementary schools in the East Harlem community of New York City, a large voluntary teaching hospital, the Mount Sinai Medical Center, provided intensive mental health and social service support for children referred by school officials for school problem behavior. The schools served are from >90% to 100% minority population, typically approximately two thirds Hispanic and one third African-American (Board of Education of the City of New York). Between 1990 and 1994, a pattern emerged: Nearly one third of children (average age, 8 years) referred for school problems lived in a household with no biological parent present. The overwhelming majority of these children were raised in a household headed by a single grandmother.

As part of mental health services, comprehensive family and social histories were obtained. Integral to these histories were inventories of social and environmental stress factors which the child and family may have experienced, including death of close family members, domestic violence, parental substance abuse, and child maltreatment. Parents or kinship caregivers were asked about prenatal drug exposure; no efforts were made to obtain birth records to verify responses. Because of the large number of children served who lived in a household with no biological parent present, funding was obtained for a comprehensive intergenerational program serving grandparent caregivers and their families, the Mount Sinai Grandparent Caregivers Program. Services included social work, counseling and support groups, legal assistance and advocacy for the grandparents, and comprehensive primary health care for the children. The program was unique in providing health care for the grandparent caregivers. Advocacy included assistance obtaining interventions for children with special needs, resolving custody issues, and ensuring receipt of health insurance benefits. All services, including adult health care, were provided at the elementary school sites.

Two studies are used to illustrate the problems experienced by children in kinship care. The first study presents data derived from a study of 170 children referred for school problems, of whom 44 (25.9%) were in kinship foster care (an additional 3.5% were in foster boarding homes, for a total of 29.4% not living with a biological parent). This was a referred population; that is, all of the children were identified as having school problems by their teachers or school administrators. These problems were confirmed by the school-based health center social service and mental health team. Excluded from this study were children of families referred to the Grandparent Caregivers Program with a referring problem or reason other than school problems.

Study two data are descriptive of children in kinship households who were referred because of their household configuration and the grandparent caregiver's need for support services. This provides a more generalized view of the incidence of special needs children in kinship households, at least in this high risk, low income community. Data are also presented on the reasons that the child was placed in kinship care, and the health status of the grandparent caregivers.

In both studies, data were derived from a detailed intake form which was completed by a social worker during an interview with the grandparent caregiver. For the first study, the school problem study, child behavioral symptoms were coded (yes/no) based on multiple classroom observations as well as interviews with the grandparents and teachers. Many of the children were also known through delivery of individual or group psychotherapy by a program social worker. Consistency of coding was maintained through ongoing meetings and further confirmed through objective observations. Diagnostic standards were overseen by a clinical child psychologist who supervised the social workers. The standard for coding "yes" for stressors and symptoms (examples, whether there was child abuse, whether behavior is considered "hyperactive") were high; that is, "neglect" might constitute the child having been left in a supermarket, and "abuse" serious physical injury. Behavior coded as "hyperactive" met American Psychiatric Association criteria consistent with the diagnosis of attention deficit hyperactivity disorder (ADHD) (APA, 1994). "Teenage mothers" were age 16 or under at the birth of their first child.

The purposes of the first study were to highlight the behavioral symptoms associated with various social and environmental stressors, to note the overlapping symptomatology and issues of co-morbidity for the diagnostic categories in common use as defined in the American Psychiatric Association *Diagnostic and Statistical Manual IV*, and to highlight the degree to which significant differential diagnostic issues may be confused or missed.

The purpose of the second study was to describe the issues affecting children and grandparents in kinship households. We were concerned that grandparent caregivers may neglect their own needs, including health care for serious chronic conditions, prioritizing the needs of the children. We therefore explored both the service needs of the grandchildren and the health status of the grandparent caregivers.

RESULTS, STUDY ONE: CHILDREN WITH SCHOOL PROBLEMS

The following demographic information applies to the 170 children referred for school problems (Grant, & Kucera, 1998):

Race/Ethnicity. Of the children referred, 105 (61.8%) were Hispanic; 60 (35.3%) were African-American, and 5 (2.9%) were "other." This essentially mirrors the racial and ethnic composition of the schools served. The distribution by sex was male, 98 (57.6%) and female 72 (42.4%). The mean age of the referred children was 7.9 years, and the mean grade was second.

Among children in kinship care, 22 (50%) were Hispanic, 21 (47.7%) were African-American, and 1 (2.3%) was "other." The mean age was 7.4 years, and the mean grade, second.

Symptoms. Data from the total sample and the subset of children in kinship care, with applicable *DSM-IV* diagnoses, are summarized in Table 1. More than one-third of the children with school problems met diagnostic criteria for each of these diagnoses: attention deficit hyperactivity disorder (ADHD), oppositional-defiant disorder, or depression. Especially striking is the co-morbidity. Among children in kinship care, five (11.4%) met criteria for both ADHD and depression; 9 (20.5%) met criteria for both ADHD and opposi-tional-defiant disorder, and 8 (18.2%) could be diagnosed with both opposi-tional-defiant disorder and depression.

Social and Environmental Stressors. For each child in the sample, social and environmental stressors affecting the family were recorded. For children in kinship care, these stressors were also the reason they were removed from their biological parents' care (e.g., abuse, death of a parent, prenatal drug exposure). Stressors for the full school problem sample and the kinship care subset are summarized in Table 2. Parental substance abuse affected three fourths of the families and was in most cases related to other stressors, including neglect and abandonment, HIV, incarceration, and death of the parent(s). Significantly correlated to kinship care placement are parental substance abuse, prenatal drug exposure, neglect/abandonment, parental HIV/AIDS ($p < 0.01$), and parental incarceration ($p < 0.05$).

TABLE 1. Symptoms of children referred for school problems.

Symptom/diagnosis	Total sample (n = 170)		Kinship subset (n = 44)	
poor concentration	103	[59.9%]	29	[65.9%]
hyperactivity	67	[9.4%]	20	[45.5%]
temper tantrums	63	[37.1%]	18	[40.9%]
mood swings	54	[31.4%]	14	[31.8%]
social isolation	14	[8.2%]	1	[2.3%]
oppositional-defiant disorder*	72	[42.4%]	16	[36.4%]
depression*	59	[34.7%]	17	[38.6%]
ADHD*	56	[32.9%]	16	[36.4%]

*American Psychiatric Association *DSM-IV* diagnostic criteria met

TABLE 2. Social and environmental stressors.

Stressor	Total sample (n = 170)		Kinship subset (n = 44)	
parental substance abuse	70	[41.2%]	34	[74.3%]
exposure to violence	55	[32.4%]	13	[29.5%]
recent death in family	42	[24.7%]	14	[31.8%]
teen mother	40	[23.5%]	9	[20.5%]
prenatal drug exposure	37	[21.8%]	23	[52.3%]
parent incarcerated	33	[19.2%]	13	[29.5%]
neglect or abandonment	30	[17.6%]	18	[40.9%]
history of homelessness	25	[14.7%]	4	[9.1%]
family history of HIV/AIDS	14	[8.2%]	8	[18.2%]

RESULTS, STUDY TWO: GRANDPARENT CAREGIVERS

Data Sources. A total of 91 kinship families comprise the sample for social and environmental stressors (Grant, Gordon, & Cohen, 1997). Health care was available to all family members in each of these 91 households; however, only 65 of the 91 kinship heads of household requested these services. Data are derived from detailed intake forms (which itemize social and environmental stressors), and a health status questionnaire, based on the Mount Sinai Hospital Internal Medicine ambulatory care intake form. Each was completed in the context of an interview with a social worker. Physical examinations, and to the extent possible review of prior medical records, were provided for the grandparents receiving health care services by either a physician's assistant or a nurse practitioner working under the direction of an internist.

Demographics. In the total sample, 62.8% of the families were Hispanic, and 37.3 African-American. The mean age of the kinship caregivers was 57.4 years with a range 35-83 years. The youngest grandparent in the program was 42; four younger maternal aunts aged 35-39 participated in the program. Four of five (80.1%) of the kinship heads of household were unmarried. All but one were women. The average household size was five individuals, including parents of the grandparent caregivers (great grandparents), other children (aunts and uncles of the children in kinship care), grandchildren (mean, 2.4 per household), and great grandchildren.

Social and Environmental Stressors/Reasons for Kinship Care. In nearly all cases, the grandparent heading the household was the biological mother's mother. Prior to kinship care, nearly all of the households had been headed by a single mother. The reasons why the child came into the grandparents' care are summarized in Table 3. For nearly two thirds of the children, substance abuse led to the parent's eventual abandonment of the child or children. Sometimes the grandparent was already a major caregiver because of the parent's unreliability.

Substance abuse was a factor in all of the parental incarcerations. By report of the grandparent, each case of mother's HIV and AIDS was due to sexual contact with an intravenous drug user who was HIV positive. The city child protection agency was involved in more than half (56%) of the cases, but these were not all formal kinship foster care placements made through Family Court. In 11% of families, the mother of the child was in jail, and the grandparent was designated as an interim caregiver until her release. Among the families where the grandparent was providing care because the biological parent had died, more than half of the deaths were due to homicide or suicide. In 15.4% of cases, the biological parent was not a competent caregiver because she was a very young teenager or was too severely mentally ill or had an intellectual disability.

Health Status of the Grandparent Caregivers. Of the 65 kinship caregivers who requested health services, 60% were Hispanic, and 40% African-American. The median age was 53.5 years. Excluding the four younger aunts from the sample, the mean age of the grandparent caregivers is 57.5 years, with a range from 42 to 78. Compared to the total sample of 91 households, Hispanic kinship caregivers were more likely to request health care services. They were also more likely to be without health insurance when they enrolled in our program.

The most pressing health care need presented was for management of chronic conditions. Many grandparents had been diagnosed with a chronic

TABLE 3. How the children came into kinship care (n = 91).

stressor	Number/percent of households
parental substance abuse, abandonment	58 [63.7%]
substantiated cases of abuse & neglect	51 [56.0%]
death of a parent	14 [15.4%]
parent incompetent, young teen, MI, ID	14 [15.4%]
parental incarceration	10 [11.0%]
parental HIV/AIDS	7 [7.7%]

condition but had not received any care, including prescribed medications, for up to ten years. A major barrier to care was inability to pay for prescription medications, especially for those grandparent caregivers covered by Medicare.

The percent of kinship caregivers (including those in their 30's) diagnosed with chronic conditions exceeded expectations based on established prevalence data (see Table 4). For example, the estimated prevalence of diabetes for adults 45-64, with household incomes less than $10,000, is 13.9%. In our comparable population, 26.2% were diabetic. Similarly, the prevalence of asthma is 10.2%; in our population it was 24.6%. Prevalence of hypertension in this age and income level is 35.7%, compared with 53.8% in our program (U.S. Centers for Disease Control, 1995). Only 16.9% of the kinship caregivers were not diagnosed with a chronic condition, and more than two thirds (67.7%) were diagnosed with multiple conditions.

Summarizing the data for the 61 grandparents only (excluding the four younger aunts), there is little variation in these frequencies. 57.4% were diagnosed with hypertension; 52.5% with arthritis; 27.9% with cardiac conditions; 26.2% with diabetes; 24.6% with asthma; 24.6% with anemia. More than two thirds, 68.9% had multiple chronic health conditions, and only 14.8% had no diagnosed chronic condition.

While this is a small sample for subset analysis of specific conditions by race and ethnicity (39 Hispanic, 26 African-American), several trends emerged. African-Americans were more likely to be diagnosed with hypertension (65.4% vs. 46.2%) while Hispanics were more likely to be diagnosed with diabetes (35.9% vs. 10.3%) and anemia (25.6% vs. 19.2%). The other conditions were more evenly distributed.

Obesity was not specifically screened, but was notable in the population. Among the grandparent caregivers, general dietary habits were very poor, characterized by high fat, high cholesterol, low protein meals. Several of the grandparents were morbidly obese; one required assistance to leave her apartment. Lack of exercise was apparent when we introduced, for social reasons, walks around the community. Many participants had difficulty walking several blocks without becoming short of breath.

Special Needs of the Children in Kinship Care. Children were designated as "special needs" if the child met eligibility criteria for developmental intervention or special education services. These criteria are established at the city and state levels based on the federal Individuals With Disabilities Education Act. Assessments and interventions were arranged through the Early Intervention Program, preschool special education, school age special education, or out-patient clinics (for psychotherapy, speech-language therapy, physical therapy, etc.).

Among these kinship households, 60.4% did not have a special needs child in residence. Nearly one third, 29.7%, had one special needs child, 5.5% had two, and 4.4% had three. Most of these children were under five years of age. The diagnoses among these children included cerebral palsy, pervasive developmental disorder, serious emotional disturbance, and intellectual disability.

DISCUSSION

As noted previously, the prevalence of special needs in a foster care population is known to be high. Kinship care is a specific kind of foster care, in which the foster parent is a family member. However, the reasons that children enter kinship care are generally the same as those which lead to a child being removed from the family into foster care. Issues such as abuse, neglect, and death of a parent frequently have a negative impact on child development and school performance. The high prevalence of special needs children revealed in these data is therefore within expectations.

Data from the school problem study reveal a high percentage of prenatally drug exposed children in kinship care. Many of these children were born between 1988 and 1992, a period in New York City when babies born to women who delivered without prenatal care (and for a period of time all babies delivered at municipal hospitals) were tested for drug exposure by urinalysis. Positive toxicology led to automatic removal of the child from the custody of the biological mother. Most often, the child was placed with a grandparent. This policy subsequently changed, and other evidence of abuse or neglect were required for the infant to be removed into any kind of foster placement.

TABLE 4. Chronic conditions of the kinship caregivers.

diagnosed chronic condition	Number/percent of caregivers	
none	11	[16.9%]
multiple diagnosed conditions	44	[67.7%]
hypertension	35	[53.8%]
arthritis	33	[50.8%]
cardiac conditions	18	[27.7%]
diabetes	17	[26.2%]
asthma	16	[24.6%]
anemia	15	[23.1%]

Consistent with the literature, caring for special needs children was a significant source of stress to the grandparent caregivers. Complaints from teachers were frequent. Referrals for special education or other interventions led grandparents into service delivery systems which were perceived as overwhelming and difficult to navigate. The burden of caring for young children who require an unusually high degree of supervision or special care contributed to the grandparents' neglect of their own health care needs. A frequent pattern emerged in that once appropriate plans for special care for the children were established, the grandparents would then focus on personal issues including health care.

In several cases ongoing therapy for a child was interrupted when care shifted from the biological parent to the grandparent, because of lost health insurance (Medicaid). There was the omnipresent risk that the special needs of the children in kinship care would not be adequately taken into account when custody decisions were made. Consistent and strong advocacy was required to keep Family Court judges aware of the nature and implications of conditions affecting the children in kinship care, so appropriate custody and visitation decisions could be made. Examples included babies with special handling requirements known to the grandparent but not the mother, and children diagnosed with autism for whom a change of custody had to be very carefully considered based on this condition.

In traditional foster care, the non-familial foster parent receives a predictable monthly subsidy to provide for the child, and the subsidy is increased if the child has special care requirements. Among grandparent caregivers who were formally designated as foster parents, non-receipt of subsidies was ubiquitous. If subsidies were received, there was resistance to increasing the rate to that which was supposed to be provided for children with special care requirements. This greatly increased the economic stress on the grandparent caregivers, sometimes compromising nutrition and access to health care when out-of-pocket expenses would be incurred (e.g., prescription medication for those covered by Medicare).

In kinship care, there are generally fewer changes in placement than in traditional foster care. Custody is likely to either remain with the relative or be restored to the parent, and the child is likely to remain in his community of origin (without disrupting pre-existing school placement and health care arrangements). However, we observed frequent tension between the biological parent and the kinship caregiver resulting in instability and conflict affecting the child. This was especially noted for children of parents who had been incarcerated.

Our assumption that the grandparents or other relatives focus on the child's needs and may therefore neglect their own was corroborated by our direct service experience. In planning interventions for kinship households, it was clear that before attempting to address problems affecting the adults, assuming they are not emergent, it was necessary first to provide concrete assistance with problems affecting the child. This not only built a trusting relationship and established the value of the provider and program, it alleviated a major source of stress on the grandparent and as such was an important intervention for the adult. The data indicate that children in kinship households may be very difficult to manage, showing signs of attention deficit disorder, conduct disorder, and depression. Counseling on discipline, limit setting, and other aspects of parenting were important services, as were providing or arranging psychotherapy for the child. It was only after teacher complaints subsided, and special education or other service needs were resolved that the grandparents would focus on more personal issues.

It is especially notable that the level of health care need of some of the grandparent caregivers was urgent, yet no efforts to obtain medical care were made until our program offered the services in a convenient community-based setting. Our program preceded mandatory participation in managed care Medicaid recipients in New York City, and it is not clear what impact, if any, the health maintenance model will have on the high level of dissatisfaction expressed (in several focus groups) by the grandparents about the health care delivery system.

Some of the immediate health care needs of the grandparents were addressed through a series of health education workshops, focusing on nutrition, and concrete activities such as walks in the community. We addressed nutritional issues through a combination of education and shopping trips–modeling how to purchase nutritious food in local markets on a tight budget.

Our data raise several questions that should be elucidated through further study. First, we found that the externalizing behavior problems of children in kinship households may indicate other psychiatric diagnoses, specifically post traumatic stress disorder and depression. Many of the prior studies cited rely on school records or questionnaires rather than direct clinical interview. A broad based study of the clinical diagnoses affecting children in foster care, based on delivery of mental health services rather than retrospective analysis of records, would be important in future service planning for this very needy population.

Second, our data on the health status of grandparent caregivers is unique in that it is based on physical examination and review of health history and records rather than self-report. The data show an unusually high rate of chronic conditions among grandparent caregivers including diabetes and hypertension. Normative data were taken from national prevalence rates based on age and income level. It is not clear whether our data are high because these are custodial grandparents (which would be consistent with prior studies) or whether the normative data for the age and income are low when applied to high risk-inner city communities such as East Harlem in New York City. It would be very important to gather appropriate prevalence data specific to high social risk populations, especially as mandatory managed care for Medicaid recipients becomes more widespread. A better understanding of the chronic conditions and specialist care needs of low income children and adults would be important to any managed care organization moving into the Medicaid market.

RECOMMENDATIONS FOR SOCIAL WORKERS

Kinship care, especially grandparent caregiving, has emerged as an alternative to foster boarding homes outside of the family. Many of the children in kinship care have been removed, formally or informally, from the care of their biological parent(s) for reasons similar to those that lead children to be placed in foster care: child abuse, neglect, abandonment, death of a parent. These factors which lead to kinship placement also may have an impact on the development, learning, and behavior of the child.

Young children in kinship care may have special needs and require services through the Early Intervention Program or preschool special education. Older children and youth in kinship care may present hyperactive and disruptive behavior in school. Programs that provide services to children with school problems, such as school-based health centers, should be prepared to provide support services for kinship caregivers. Similarly, programs that serve grandparent and other kinship caregivers should be prepared to provide or arrange interventions for their special needs children.

While the behavioral profile of many of the children in kinship care is suggestive of a diagnosis of ADHD or a conduct disorder, these symptom-based diagnoses may miss underlying problems such as depression or post-traumatic stress disorder. A detailed social history should be taken for any child in kinship care with school problems. The reasons why the child entered kinship care should be made known to any mental health or special education provider.

Advocacy should be integral to any program for grandparent and other kinship caregivers. This must include access to legal services for assistance with court cases involving custody, as well as benefits entitlement advocacy for health benefits, cash subsidies for child care responsibilities, special needs differentials to these subsidies, SSI payments for special needs children, etc. Special attention should be paid to custody issues affecting children with special needs.

The stresses associated with parenting a behaviorally difficult and/or special needs child exacerbate the economic and emotional stress of being in the parental role for one's grandchild. Providing interventions for the special needs child constitutes an important intervention for the kinship caregiver. Alleviating stress around the child's difficulties establishes a working relationship in which the grandparent may be more willing to discuss personal needs and problems, including unmet health care needs.

For kinship caregivers, prioritizing the needs of the children in their care was an additional barrier to obtaining health care. This was sufficiently powerful to interfere with seeking care for potentially life threatening conditions such as diabetes and hypertension. Programs that serve grandparent caregivers should screen for health problems, ensure adequate health insurance, and facilitate access to a primary health care provider. Lifelong poor nutrition and lack of exercise were serious problems in the population we served. A simple program of exercise (including short walking trips), health education, and nutrition counseling, can be extremely beneficial.

On a policy level, programs that serve young children should have procedures which are more easily navigated by grandparents and other kinship caregivers. This applies to pediatric settings as well as entitlement programs for children with disabilities. Medicare should cover the cost of prescription drugs which are medically necessary. There can be life threatening consequences for people with conditions such as diabetes and hypertension if medical care includes a prescription for medication which cannot be obtained.

REFERENCES

American Psychiatric Association. (1994). *Diagnostic and Statistical Manual of Mental Disorders, Fourth Edition (DSM-IV)*. Washington, DC: American Psychiatric Press, Inc.

Berrick, J.D. (1994). When children cannot remain home: Foster family care and kinship care. *The Future of Children, 8*, [1], 899-911.

Brockway, K. (1998). Latino grandparent caregivers found in poor health, poverty. *Columbia University Record, 23*, [16], Internet.

Brookdale Center on Aging, The Grandparent Caregiver Law Center. (1999). *www.brookdale.org/gpc*

Child Welfare League of America. (1999). *Children '99: Countdown to the Millennium Fact Sheet.*

Carnegie Corporation of New York. (1994). *Starting Points: Meeting the Needs of Our Youngest Children*. New York: Carnegie Corporation.

Emick, M.A., & Hayslip Jr., B. (1999). Custodial grandparenting: Stresses, coping skills, and relationships with grandchildren. *International Journal of Aging and Human Development, 48*, [1], 35-61.

Fuller-Thomson, E., Minkler, M., & Driver, D.A. (1997). A profile of grandparents raising grandchildren in the United States. *Gerontologist, 37*, [3], 406-411.

Grant, R., & Kucera, E. (1998). Social and environmental stressors affecting an inner city school problem population. National Assembly on School-Based Health Care.

Grant, R., Gordon, G., & Coehn, S.T. (1997). *Health status of grandparent caregivers . . . and the special needs of the children in their care.* Scientific Meeting of the Gerontological Society of America. Washington, D.C.

Halfon, N., Berkowitz, G., & Klee, L. (1992). Mental health service utilization by children in foster care in California. *Pediatrics, 89,* [6/2], 1238-1244.

Harden, A.W., Clark, R.L., & Maguire, K. (1997). *Formal and Informal Kinship Care.* Washington, DC: U.S. Department of Health and Human Services.

Kendall, K.A., & Eckenrode, J. (1996). The effects of neglect on academic achievement and disciplinary problems: A developmental perspective. *Child Abuse and Neglect, 20,* [3], 161-169.

Kurtz, P.D., Graudin, J.M., Wodarski, J.S., & Howing, P.T. (1993). Maltreatment and the school aged child: School performance consequences. *Child Abuse and Neglect, 17,* [5], 581-589.

Minkler, M., & Fuller-Thomson, E. (1999). The health of grandparents raising grandchildren: Results of a national study. *American Journal of Public Health, 89,* [9], 1384-1389.

Minkler, M. (1997). Grandparents become parents all over again. *Berkeley Magazine, 3,* [2], Internet. www.urel.berkeley.edu/UREL_1/fall_97/departments/discoveries/minkler.html

National Center for Policy Analysis. (1997). *Policy Report No. 210,* Internet. www.ncpa.org

National Committee to Preserve Social Security and Medicare. (1998). The Statistics. Washington, DC: DHHS.

Pilowsky, D. (1995). Psychopathology among children placed in foster care. *Psychiatric Services, 46,* [9], 906-910.

Runyan, D.K., & Gould, C.L. (1985). Foster care for child maltreatment. II. Impact on school performance. *Pediatrics, 76,* [5], 841-847.

Sawyer, R.J., & Dubowitz, H. (1994). School performance of children in kinship care. *Child Abuse and Neglect, 18,* [7], 587-597.

Schor, E.L. (1982). The foster care system and health status of foster children. *Pediatrics, 69,* [5], 521-528.

Simms, M.D., & Halfon, N. (1994). The health care needs of children in foster care: A research agenda. *Child Welfare, 73,* [5], 505-524.

Stanton, A.M. (1998). Grandparents' visitation rights and custody. *Child and Adolescent Psychiatric Clinics of North America, 7,* [2], 409-422.

Takayama, J.I., Bergman, A.B., & Connell, F.A. (1994). Children in foster care in the state of Washington. Health care utilization and expenditures. *Journal of the American Medical Association, 271,* [23], 1850-1855.

United States Census Bureau. (1999). www.handsnet.org

United States Centers for Disease Control, National Center for Health Statistics. (1995). *Table 60: Number of selected reported chronic conditions per 1,000 persons, by family income and age, 10,* [199]. Washington, DC: DHHS.

United States Department of Health and Human Services. (1998). *Trends in the Well-being of America's Children and Youth.* Washington, DC: DHHS.

Grandparent Caregivers I: Characteristics of the Grandparents and the Children with Disabilities for Whom They Care

Matthew P. Janicki, PhD
Philip McCallion, PhD, ACSW
Lucinda Grant-Griffin, PhD
Stacey R. Kolomer, CSW

SUMMARY. Using an informal data capture technique, 164 grandparents caring for 208 children with developmental delay or diagnosed disabilities were surveyed in New York City to determine their health status, emotional state, use of formal and informal services, and general life situation. The vast majority of grandparents were female (96%) and African-American (80%). Their ages ranged from 40 to 82. Generally they had cared for at least one grandchild for an average of seven years. The data showed that for these grandparents (1) caregiving was an all-consuming role, (2) their lives were fraught with uncertainty and they

Matthew P. Janicki is Research Professor, and Philip McCallion is Assistant Professor and Hartford Geriatric Social Work Faculty Scholar, School of Social Welfare, University at Albany. Lucinda Grant-Griffin is Policy Analyst, New York State Office of Mental Retardation and Developmental Disabilities, Albany, NY. Stacey R. Kolomer is a Doctoral Candidate associated with the Centre on Intellectual Disabilities, School of Social Welfare, University at Albany.

Address correspondence to: Matthew P. Janicki, PhD, RI 280, University at Albany, 135 Western Avenue Albany, NY 12222 (E-mail: mpjzj@aol.com).

Funding for this project was provided by the Joseph P. Kennedy, Jr., Foundation.

[Haworth co-indexing entry note]: "Grandparent Caregivers I: Characteristics of the Grandparents and the Children with Disabilities for Whom They Care." Janicki, Matthew P. et al. Co-published simultaneously in *Journal of Gerontological Social Work* (The Haworth Press, Inc.) Vol. 33, No. 3, 2000, pp. 35-55; and: *Grandparents as Carers of Children with Disabilities: Facing the Challenges* (ed: Philip McCallion and Matthew Janicki) The Haworth Press, Inc., 2000, pp. 35-55. Single or multiple copies of this article are available for a fee from The Haworth Document Delivery Service [1-800-342-9678, 9:00 a.m. - 5:00 p.m. (EST). E-mail address: getinfo@haworthpressinc.com].

35

could not access sufficient formal and informal supports, and (3) they were constantly worried about the future. *[Article copies available for a fee from The Haworth Document Delivery Service: 1-800-342-9678. E-mail address: <getinfo@haworthpressinc.com> Website: <http://www.HaworthPress.com>]*

KEYWORDS. Impact of caregiving on grandparents, special needs grandchildren, African-American grandparents, access to services

Over the past decade increasing attention has been paid to the many older families who have provided a lifetime of care to family members with disabilities. Researchers have generally described the average caregiving family as a mother in her 60-70's caring for a daughter with a disability in her 40's (Heller & Factor, 1991; Seltzer & Krauss, 1994; Smith, Fullmer & Tobin, 1994). Now, there are growing reports of older women caring for persons with developmental delays and disabilities who are children or young adults (Janicki, McCallion, Force, Bishop, & LePore, 1996). These younger family members are usually grandchildren or great grandchildren. Drug addiction, AIDS, and criminal activity have increasingly resulted in parents not being available to care for their child with a disability, and grandparents assuming this responsibility. Little is known about this population of grandparents, except that members of "multi-cultural" and inner city communities are over-represented, many grandparents are approaching service systems in crisis, and service systems are not equipped to meet grandparents' unique needs.

This article provides a preliminary picture of skip-generation caregiving of children with disabilities by describing a population of grandparent carers located in New York City, discussing their needs, identifying some of the concerns and consequences that result from caregiving, and providing recommendations for workers concerned with providing effective outreach and supports.

CHANGING CIRCUMSTANCES
AND ROLES FOR GRANDPARENTS

The number of elderly persons in the United States has almost doubled from nearly 17 million in 1960. It is projected that there will be 51.1 million elderly persons by 2020, and 66.6 million by 2040. The most rapid growth will occur among those age 85 and older (Biegel & Blum, 1990; Cantor, 1991). Older minority group members are also a rapidly growing segment of the population (Angel & Hogan, 1992; Aponte & Couch, 1995). Such persons constituted 20% of the elderly in 1980, and 26% of the elderly by 1995.

They are projected to constitute 33% of the elderly by 2050 (Markides & Miranda, 1997). However, concerns remain regarding health status indicators for African-American and Hispanic/Latino elderly adults are less healthy than their counterparts of European or Asian backgrounds (Gibson, 1991; Stump, Clark, Johnson, & Wolinsky, 1997). On other measures, African-American and Hispanic/Latino elderly have also been found to have less formal education and occupational status, are over-represented in the lower socioeconomic strata of society, and have fewer retirement resources (Nickens, 1995; Shay, Miles, & Hayward, 1996). These concerns notwithstanding, contemporary elderly adults are likely to be healthier and more affluent than in earlier generations and to experience grandparenthood and great grandparenthood extending for as long as fifty years (NIA, 1995; Shore & Hayslip, 1994).

Matching the extension in time and numbers of individuals involved in aging and grandparenting experiences, there have been also been changes in roles from the "enjoyment and pleasure" picture often associated with the retirement years (NIA, 1995). More aging persons are working outside the home (Smith, 1991). Caregiving is also increasingly a part of the aged years; including caring for frail and ill spouses (Toseland, Smith, & McCallion, 1995), adult children with disabilities who have received lifelong care from a parent (Janicki et al., 1998), and adult children returning home or requiring other assistance (Spitze & Logan, 1992). Most recently, an additional role is being recognized: care for grandchildren.

Historically, families have provided care for kin in need (Burnette, 1997). Grandparents often function as the safety net for children whose parents are unwilling or unable to care for them (Minkler, Roe, & Price, 1992). For example, during the civil war it was common for African-American grandmothers to care for their grandchildren while their children were seeking employment in the North (Burton, 1992). The Depression Era was another period when, to facilitate the search by parents for employment, grandparents frequently took responsibility for the care of their grandchildren (Mullen, 1996). Similarly, multi-generational families living in one household became common place during World War II when large numbers of men went to war and women needed assistance from their own mothers as they balanced child care and jobs. The decline in the size of families and the postponing of child bearing years probably masked the need for grandparent assistance during the more recent decades. However, the past ten years have been marked by a significant increase in the number of grandparents who are the caretakers of their grandchildren, and for reasons other than employment needs. Also, universally grandparents are becoming the exclusive carers for many of these children.

INCREASES IN THE NUMBER
OF GRANDCHILDREN NEEDING CARE

Traditionally, divorce, death, and abandonment caused small numbers of grandparents to become permanent and primary carers to their grandchildren (Pinson-Millburn, Schlossberg, & Pyle, 1996). More recently, other factors have led grandparent headed households to become more common as a type of home for children. For example, the number of child abuse and neglect reports have dramatically increased (Dubowitz, Feigelman, Harrington, Starr, & Zuravin, 1994). There was a 24 percent increase in reports of child abuse and neglect between 1985 and 1994, which now total more than three million reports each year (Kelley, Yorker, & Whiteley, 1997). Increases in the number of pregnant teenagers unprepared for parenthood, and growing instances of AIDS, homelessness, unemployment, poverty, maternal imprisonment, and, particularly, substance abuse, have also contributed to an increased inability of parents to care for their own children (Dubowitz et al., 1994; Pinson-Millburn et al., 1996).

Children living in grandparent headed homes dramatically increased between 1980 and 1994. In 1980 an estimated 2.2 million children lived in grandparent headed homes and by 1994 this had increased to between 3.7 and 3.9 million children: a 40 percent increase within a 14-year period (Burnette, 1997; Hanson & Opsahl, 1996; Mullen, 1996). In approximately one-fourth to one-third of the grandparent headed households, the child's parent was not present in the home (Flint & Perez-Porter, 1996; Karp, 1996); this represents 1.3 million children living in households without a parent present (Scannapieco, Hegar, & McAlpine, 1997) and is expected to continue to grow.

THE POSITIVE AND NEGATIVE CONSEQUENCES
OF CAREGIVING

Even though it is often demanding and stressful, caregiving is frequently perceived by aging caregivers as a rewarding experience. Rewards include greater intimacy and love, finding meaning through the experience of caregiving, personal growth, improved relationships, experiencing satisfaction, and appreciation of received social support from others (Toseland, Smith & McCallion, in press). Similar to other aging carers, some grandparents do report drawing strength from knowing that they are holding their family together (Minkler et al., 1992). Caregiving has also been reported as associated with better health among some carers (Kramer, 1997). Consistent with these general reports, some grandparents also report that their own health has improved since assuming caregiving. One such grandmother, for example, reported that upon assuming care for her granddaughter she immediately gave up smoking and as a consequence felt her own health improve (Minkler et al., 1992). However, Jendrek (1994) and Minkler and Roe (1993) warn that grandparents often over-report their well-being and satisfaction, because their most over-riding concern is that their grandchildren do not go into foster care. They agree with Miller (1991) that depression, insomnia, and hypertension are frequently present. Moreover, most studies acknowledge that even the most optimistic grandparents stated they often felt isolated, and a large percentage of grandparents reported feeling overwhelmed and depressed. This was particularly the case when they thought about the future for themselves and for their grandchildren. For example, an exploratory study by Minkler and colleagues (1992) of the physical and emotional health of 75 grandmothers caring for grandchildren born to crack cocaine-addicted mothers found that 51% percent of the grandmothers reported feeling emotionally depressed. In addition, half said they could not get going and that they were totally exhausted; a third reported feeling lonely. Yet, even among this group of grandmothers the investigators found an intense desire to keep their grandchild at home, and a willingness to deny their own symptoms and needs, lest it result in the removal of the grandchild.

In contrast to other aging carers, there are many indications that grandparents who assume care for a grandchild have a higher risk for symptoms of emotional burnout and depression. For example, Fuller-Thompson and colleagues have reported from an analysis of the National Survey of Families and Households that, compared to their age peers, caregiving grandparents are almost twice as likely to have levels of depressive symptoms above the traditional Center for Epidemiologic Studies Depression Scale (CES-D) cut off point of 16 (25% vs. 15%). Even when the authors controlled for baseline depression and demographic variables known to contribute to depressive symptoms, they found that undertaking the care of a grandchild was associated with significantly higher depressive symptoms (Minkler, Fuller-Thompson, Miller & Driver, 1997).

In addition to the act of assuming care for a grandchild, three sets of risk factors for emotional depression and other negative consequences of caregiving have been identified for grandparents. One set of risk factors encompasses *level of caregiving demands*. The greater the health concerns and other caregiving needs presented by the grandchildren, the more overwhelmed grandparents reported feeling (Burton, 1992). A second set of risk factors are focused on *parents' reasons for relinquishing care* to grandparents. The decision often results from poverty, crack cocaine usage, alcohol, AIDS, incarceration, or violence including abuse or neglect of the child. Grandparent ties to the grandchild's ill, incarcerated or addicted parent, having unresolved issues regarding the death of the child's parent, and past difficulties in the interactions of the parent with the legal and health care systems all increase stress for grandparents (Barnhill, 1996; Burton, 1992; Minkler et al., 1992). A third set of risk factors is the *absence or paucity of needed formal and informal supports.* The absence of regular and dependable respite is reported as likely to be a major concern for grandparents who are isolated, or who are facing the most demanding caregiving concerns (Burton, 1992; Minkler et al., 1992).

Conversely, having informal supports, respite, and other tangible formal services available is potentially an important protective factor for some grandparents. Many grandparent carers have identified their need for respite, a "break," as critical (Burton, 1992; Minkler et al., 1992). Because of their preoccupation with carer demands, they report feeling shunned by their own peers who have long since relinquished caregiving responsibilities and show little willingness to help them out with their carer responsibilities. This shunning increases their isolation and reduces the likelihood of relief or other informal help. The absence of regular and dependable respite is likely to be an even greater concern for grandparents who are the most isolated, i.e., those providing the most hands-on caregiving. This includes grandparents caring for children with disabilities.

CAREGIVING FOR CHILDREN WITH DISABILITIES

Many of the already listed causes of grandparent assumption of care such as abuse, neglect, and drug and alcohol abuse have long been known to also have strong linkages to causes of intellectual and developmental disabilities, psychiatric impairments, and other similar conditions. For example, tobacco and crack cocaine addiction and AIDS among parents may result in physical health problems for the children, and in developmental disorders such as attention deficit and conduct disorders, autism, and other intellectual disabilities. These problems are often confounded by premature birth, poor nutrition, and inadequate stimulation in their early years, while still under the care of their parent. Care for such children is also likely to be more demanding than care for children without disabilities. Yet, there has been little consideration in the existing literature of grandparents caring for children with disabilities. A possible explanation is offered by Kolomer (2000) who reports that grandparents caring for a child with a disability who become kinship foster care providers are usually expected to fit into existing foster care services with few additional supports. They become part of a generic group of special needs children that also includes sibling groups, older children, and children of minority groups. The existing literature on grandparent carers, whether they are formal or informal carers, does not consider the uniqueness of caring for a child with a disability. Not being identified as a unique group, their specific needs and experiences have not been considered and are often over-looked.

Other literature does indicate that caring for a person with a disability and its consequences for the caregiver are different from other caregiving experiences. For example, care for a child with a disability by parents has been reported to be often more difficult than other types of parenting, because of the consequences of emotional strains, sibling conflicts, difficult developmental transitions, increased financial burdens, restructuring of family roles and deferral of career goals, particularly by the mother (for a review, see McCallion & Toseland, 1993), and having to deal with specialty educational, medical and social service agencies not normally encountered in children without these difficulties. The literature also cites many rewards. This appears particularly true for older parental caregivers who have offered a lifetime of care to now adult sons and daughters. They have been reported to be resilient, optimistic, and healthier than non-caregiving women their own age (Krauss & Seltzer, 1993). However, the experience of caring for young children with a disability in one's later years places different demands than caring earlier in one's life. Also, grandmothers now assuming a caregiving role will usually not have the benefits of a lifetime's experience of caregiving for an individual with a disability, to which Seltzer and Krauss (1994) attach importance in explaining their findings for older carers. Reliance on existing literature and research findings is not enough. Given the important developmental needs of young children with disabilities, and the mounting evidence of risks for emotional depression and other health consequences for grandparents assuming care, it is important that the experiences and consequences of grandparents assuming care for children with disabilities be fully explored.

METHOD

Participants

The study involved 164 grandparents residing in two of New York City's five boroughs, who were caring for at least one child with a developmental delay or disability. Recruitment involved two methods and occurred over a 15 month period during 1998-1999. The first recruitment effort involved three community based local service agencies serving the Queens and Bronx boroughs of New York City. Representatives of these agencies were asked to locate grandparents living in their catchment areas who were caring for at least one child with a developmental delay or disability. They used a variety of outreach methods, including posting notices at churches, hairdressing salons, convenience stores and bodegas, health centers and human service agencies. They also employed word of mouth recruitment through local churches, cultural community organizations, and participant grandparents. This first method resulted in 88 participants. The second recruitment effort involved drawing from grandparent carers who called into a telephone hot-line for grandparent concerns operated by the New York City Department for the Aging's Grandparent Resource Center. Grandparents who called in over a 12-month period were asked if they would like to participate in a telephone survey and, if they did, were recruited for the study. This resulted in an additional 76 grandparents.

Instrument

A specially developed interview protocol contained both project-specific items and several standardized questionnaires. The specially developed inter-view protocol was used as the main instrument. Pre-testing of the protocol involved using a focus group of ten grandparents. During discussions with the focus group, several instruments originally considered for use were found to be difficult to administer over the telephone and were replaced with more productive alternatives. In addition, wording and meaning problems were identified and clarified, and the validity of the issues being researched were established. Originally participants were expected to meet the typical grand-parent profile (skip generation, related adult in his/her 60s or older). The focus group pointed out that "grandparents" may be a variety of related or unrelated adults (e.g., the second wife of a biological grandfather; a friend/ neighbor who has functioned in this role; a great aunt; or a great grandpar-ent). Thus, for the purposes of the study, "grandparent carer" was defined as "an individual who has assumed primary care for the individual, is at least one generation removed for the child's own parent(s), and perceives him/her-self in a grandparenting relationship with the child."

The focus group also helped in pointing out questions that may pose difficulties for grandparents to answer, and offered strategies for interviewers to put grandparents at ease. The final instrument was a 210 item protocol (which is available from the senior author upon request). It was used in both an English and Spanish form. A backward and forward translation process was used to ensure compatibility between the two forms. Two independent translators were used. One translator was a community leader working with grandparents who also ensured that the translations of the measures were culturally and linguistically appropriate (Zambrana, 1991).

The protocol contained questions related to both the grandparents and the children/adults in the home. With regard to the grandparents, data included demographics (such as age, sex, education, ethnicity, religion, marital status, employment and number of children under care). Care-related questions included reasons for assuming care, how long they expected to be the carer, who would assume care when they were no longer able, other caregiving responsibilities, contact with children's parents, and service need and use.

Standardized Instruments. Grandparent health status was measured using four dimensions of health drawn from the Medical Outcomes Study Short Form Health Survey (SF20; Stewart, Hays, & Ware, 1988). The dimensions were: health perceptions, physical functioning, role functioning, and social functioning. Higher scores on health perception suggest better perceived health, and lower scores on the other three subscales suggest increased limitation as a result of their perceived health concerns. The subscales have been shown to have good reliability and validity (Hays & Stewart, 1990). Symptoms of depression among grandparents were assessed using the Center for Epidemiologic Studies Depression Scale (CES-D; Radloff, 1977). The CES-D was selected because it has been used widely, has a cut off score suggestive of depression, and offers opportunities to compare findings with other studies of grandparent carers (Fuller-Thompson et al., 1997; Radloff, 1977). Finally, grandparents' sense of caregiving mastery was measured using a 7-item scale developed by Pearlin and Schooler (1978). The scale measures generalized expectations about one's ability to influence events in life using a four point agree/disagree format (Huyck, 1991). It was previously found to have good reliability when used with older caregivers of diverse ethnicity (Pruchno, Patrick, & Burant, 1997). Some wording changes were made so that items addressed grandparent carers.

A generic service-utilization survey was so used. Grandparents were asked to assess their need for, and use of a listing of 15 formal services such as respite, day programs, and transportation which the pre-test group had identified as particularly helpful to grandparent carers.

Children's Data. A specially developed data form collected primary information regarding the children, including the child's age and sex, legal status and responsibility for care, and diagnoses. The focus group had suggested that young children in grandparent care may not yet have a formal diagnosis, although disabilities may be present. Because it was also noted that some grandparents are reluctant to have their grandchildren examined by health clinics or child study teams, eight questions regarding the child's behavior were included (drawn from a previous study describing developmental delays and disabilities–Janicki et al., 1996).

Data Collection

Interviewers were trained by the principal investigator and were usually of the same ethnic and cultural background as the grandparent respondents; several were grandparent carers. In most instances, interviews were conducted by telephone. When grandparents preferred a personal interview, they were interviewed in person. Most interviews took from 45 to 90 minutes to complete. Some lasted as long as four hours because the grandparents used the interview as an opportunity to talk about their experiences in a way that they were unable to with family and others. Because of the length of the protocol, grandparents were given the option of completing the interview in one or more telephone or personal contacts. Several interviews were broken down into 5-6 segments because caregiving needs did not give the grandparents sufficient free time to complete the protocol in one session.

RESULTS

The vast majority of caregiving grandparents were female (96%) and African-American (80%), and had an average age of 60 (range 40 to 82; *s.d.* = 8.94). As indicated on Table 1, some 30% had an available spouse, 29% were educated beyond high school, and 26% were also holding a job. They have lived in New York City for an average of 45 years (range 2-74 years; *s.d.* = 14.6) and cared for a grandchild for an average of seven years (range 1-35; *s.d.* = 5.4). Most were caring for one or two grandchildren ($X = 1.9$; *s.d.* = 1.4).

There are a variety of reasons why the grandparents assumed care (Table 2). Substance abuse by the child's parent was the primary reason (44%), with preventing placement of the child in foster care as the second most prevalent (20%). Grandparents reported that the risk of foster care placement usually resulted from parental child abuse and neglect concerns. A majority of grandparents expected to care for the children until they were able to care for themselves and hoped that another relative would assume care if they were no longer able. A relatively small number (12%) had expectations that the child's parent would reclaim the responsibility of caregiving. About a quarter reported having no idea how long they would have to provide care, or not knowing who would assume their responsibilities if they were no longer able to continue to provide care. Less than 1% was prepared to consider the possibility that foster care agencies would assume care. About 40% had additional responsibilities for caring for someone else besides their grandchildren, usually a parent or spouse with a chronic illness, or their own adult child with a disability, or mental health or substance abuse problem.

Most maintained contact with the child's parents, usually with the mother. Some 57% reported at least weekly contacts; however, they reported that such contacts were not always helpful. For example, the natural parents often made promises to the children that they would stop using drugs, or would provide a home again for the child that they were not able to fulfill. Grandparents also reported that their attempts to set rules for the grandchildren were often undermined by parents' gifts and indulgences designed to make up for their absence. They also reported difficulties in barring the parents

TABLE 1. Grandparent Demographics (n = 164)

Age	
≤ 59	52%
60-69	35%
≤ 70	13%
Sex	
Female	96%
Male	4%
Ethnicity	
African American	80%
European	7%
Hispanic/Latino	9%
Native American	2%
Other	2%
Religion	
Catholic	15%
Jewish	1%
Protestant	84%
Marital Status	
Married/Live-in Relationship	30%
Divorced/Separated	26%
Widowed	32%
Never Married	12%
Education	
Some High School	33%
High School Graduate	37%
Some College	22%
College Graduate	7%
Work	
Grandparent Employed	26%
Housing Situation	
Rents	62%
Owns	38%

from the home, and a desire not to alienate the grandchildren from their natural parents.

Grandparents reported using few of the 15 formal services, such as case management, assistance with housing issues and support groups, which the pre-test group had identified as particularly helpful to grandparent carers. Although they reported generally using only one or two of the services (range: 0-12; $X = 1.44$, *s.d.* = 2.12), they reported needing four or five (range: 0-15; $X = 4.63$; *s.d.* = 4.42).

As noted in Table 3, grandparents tended to report high perceptions of

TABLE 2. Grandparent Caregiving Circumstances (n = 164)

Reason for assuming care		Continued contact with parent	
Parent died	8%	No, deceased	8%
Parent using drugs	44%	No, in jail	3%
Parent in jail	12%	Yes, with both parents	20%
Parent has AIDS	1%	Yes, with mother only	61%
Parent hospitalized	3%	Yes, with father only	8%
Parent out of area	11%		
To prevent placement of child		**Frequency of parental contact**	
in foster care	20%	Daily	20%
		Weekly	37%
How long does grandparent expect		Monthly	14%
to care for grandchildren		1-2 times per year	6%
Until able to care for selves	54%	Irregular	22%
Will always be the carer	8%		
Until son/daughter gets	12%	Also caring for other	
better		family members	40%
Don't know how long	27%		
Who will care when grandparent is no longer able:			
Mother/father of child	19%		
Another relative	56%		
Foster care	>1%		
Don't know who	24%		

their overall health and a low level of limitations on physical and role functioning. To provide some perspective, their scores on the MOS-20 were compared to scores reported for a study of aging spousal caregivers of persons with chronic illness (Toseland, O'Donnell, Engelhardt, Richie, Jue, & Banks, 1997). The spousal caregivers reported poorer health and greater health limitations. However, reported limitations on grandparent social functioning appeared high when compared to spousal caregiver reports (2.18 compared to 4.08) and suggest the presence of limitations most of the time. Grandparent responses also indicated an average score of 17.19 on the CES-D, i.e., more than 50% report a level of symptoms suggesting clinical depres-

TABLE 3. Grandparent Health and Psychological Status

Variable	Mean	SD
Health (MOS-20)	16.98	3.76
Health perceptions	3.71	2.07
Physical functioning	1.16	0.94
Role functioning		
Social functioning	2.18	1.53
Psychological		
Depressive symptoms (CES-D)	17.19	10.24
Caregiving mastery (Pearlin)	20.49	3.10

sion. Finally, the mean score of 20.49 on the caregiving mastery scale suggests that grandparents did feel somewhat in control of their lives (the range of possible scores was from a low of 7 to a high of 28).

Grandchild Findings. Two hundred and eight grandchildren were being cared for by the 164 grandparent carers in the sample (X = 1.26 children per household). As shown in Table 4, 59% of the children were male; their average age was 11 years (*s.d.* = 4.83; range 1-53). However, within the sample there were 18 children with disabilities over age 18, of whom 10 were over age 21, the usual age for termination of special education services. The presence of these older care recipients in the group masks the fact that many of the children cared for were infants, toddlers, and primary grade age. At the other end of the range, it should be noted that some grandparents had been primary carers of adult grandchildren with disabilities for up to 35 years. Most grandparents (86%) reported that they had legal responsibility for their grandchildren, but actual legal status ranged from legal adoption (9%) to kinship foster care (14%) to on-going court involvement in establishing status (62%) to informal care (14%).

Table 4 shows that many of the children had received formal diagnoses through their schools and health clinics. Multiple problems or handicaps had been identified for 60% of the sample, intellectual and other developmental disabilities were established for 53% and learning problems and attention deficit and hyperactivity disorders were a diagnosis for 52% and 34% respectively. Grandparents were also asked to indicate if a number of behaviors were present for their grandchildren as a way of identifying delays and disabilities not yet receiving formal diagnosis. Some 76% reported problems

TABLE 4. Grandchild Demographics (n = 208)

Age	
< 5	10%
5-9	32%
10-14	35%
15-19	18%
20+	4%
Gender	
Female	41%
Male	59%
Diagnosis given to grandparents	
Multiple problems	60%
Learning problems	52%
Attention deficit hyperactivity disorder	34%
Developmental disability	31%
Intellectual disability	22%
Vision or hearing impaired	16%
Neurologically impaired	13%
Autism	6%
Speech problems	6%
Epilepsy	5%
Cerebral palsy	4%
Legal responsibility for child	
Grandparent	86%
Parent	11%
Other	3%
Grandparent description of children's problems	
Problems in school	76%
Behaviors that are difficult to control	63%
Child not able to do things children of same age can do	61%
Other people having more than expected difficulty understanding child	44%
Health problems	41%
Problems hearing and/or seeing	24%
Problems walking	20%
Problems holding things	14%
Legal status of child	
Grandparent, court appointed guardian	37%
Grandparent, temporary court custody	20%
Kinship foster care	14%
Informal care	14%
Legally adopted by grandparent	9%
Being established	5%

in school, 63% were concerned about behaviors that were difficult to control, and 61% stated that their grandchild was not able to do things that other children of their age were able to do.

DISCUSSION

Skip-generation caregiving is a phenomenon that has lately received a great deal of attention. One aspect that has been generally overlooked is the caregiving by grandparents caring for children with disabilities. This study queried 164 grandparents in such a caregiving role. The data from this subset of grandparent carers, led us to observe that in many instances such grandparents face the same challenges as do other grandparent carers, but at other times their challenges are unique. Similarities occur in how they are challenged by their responsibilities and by fearing that they will be perceived as inadequate in their roles. Perceived differences revolved around the realities of often being overwhelmed by the nature of their grandchild's disabilities. Generally, we observed that (1) caregiving was an all-consuming role in their lives, (2) their days were fraught with uncertainty because they generally could not access sufficient formal and informal supports, and (3) they were constantly worried about remaining alive long enough to provide care for their grandchildren into adulthood.

A key finding in our study was that these grandparents, like others who are carers, expressed a high level of concern over how they were perceived with regard to their caregiving role. While most inherited their grandchildren because of their own child's incapacity or inability to parent, and a concern that the grandchild may end up in foster care, the grandparents were also driven by worries that public authorities may deem them incapable and proceed to take their grandchildren from them. This perception was compounded by feelings of being aged and overwhelmed, and of often being at odds with society's perceptions of who takes care of young children. A further factor was that their grandchild may have a recognizable disability that required special attention. Thus, they often tried to present a picture of good health and capability to ensure that they were perceived as capable, at least to public authorities. For example, when queried about their health, most reported being in good health and having few health related limitations—generally, they reported a better health status and having fewer limitations than age-equivalent peers caring for spouses with chronic illness. However, as has been found by others (Jendrek, 1994; Minkler & Roe, 1993), we observed that global questions asking grandparents about their health probably often result in overly positive responses. Yet, more focused questions or observations on their day-to-day lives and interactions often resulted in greater acknowledgment of limitations. For example, during the pre-test focus group, a number of participating grandparents stated that they were in good-to-excellent health, yet, this was not validated by personal observations. One meeting was delayed when two grandparents appeared winded and asked for time to slow heart palpitations after they had climbed to the third floor when the meeting was held.

In our survey population, the grandparents related concerns about others seeing them as not being able to care for their grandchildren. (In contrast, this is not a concern generally highlighted among older adults caring for a spouse or an aged parent.) Thus, many masked their day-to-day difficulties so as not to give the impression that they could not continue to provide care. Yet, to the extent that older age is associated with higher risks for chronic illness and other infirmities, grandparents caring for children with disabilities do have health needs. Further, findings that these grandparent carers may exaggerate their own good health, and are reluctant to acknowledge their health needs should lead workers to pay greater attention to this issue. Proffering non-judgmental assistance with meeting their own health needs and helping to provide linkages to appropriate health practitioners would go far in alleviating many of the health related concerns that such grandparents may experience.

A second finding was that care for children with disabilities is demanding and as a consequence, the grandparents' lives are fraught with uncertainty for they were often unable to access sufficient formal and informal supports. Having to provide care for children with serious behavioral difficulties or cognitive and/or physical disabilities was the differentiating factor between these grandparents and other grandparent carers with less stressful or de-manding lives. The fact that over three-quarters of the grandparents reported that the children they care for had problems in school and that two-thirds were concerned about behaviors that they found difficult to control was telling. Indeed, some 60% of children in our sample were reported to have behavioral or physical conditions that were complex and coincident. Many of the grandparents reported never being able to leave their grandchild alone or with someone else, experiencing disrupted sleep, having physical challenges (such as having to carry the child up and down many stairs), and being physically assaulted. Although acknowledging the help they often received from spouses, their own children, and local agencies, the grandparents gener-ally expressed a need for even more supports, but had difficulty obtaining the services they really needed.

In addition, they often reported that they had difficulty accessing services because of ambiguous guardianship and legal situations, were frustrated by time-consuming appointments and regulatory hurdles, and feared acknowl-edging needs might result in removal of the child. They continued to worry about their own ability to provide care over the long term as the child got older and disabilities became more obvious. Such situations should be a signal for workers to reach out to these families rather than wait for them to seek services. In such instances, outreach and service delivery should be nonjudgmental and focused on supporting families rather than finding fault.

The grandparents in our cohort acknowledged focusing more on their grandchildren's needs rather than thinking about themselves. This degree of child-centered commitment often had social and personal consequences. Many found that they were excluded from peer activities and could not enjoy the fruits of their own old age, as could their friends who were not carers (such as missed card games, trips out of the City, social events, and times spent at the senior center). The grandparents acknowledged limitations in their ability to engage in social activities. This is consistent with grandparents' verbal reports of never having time for themselves and the things they like to do, and the isolation they experienced with few opportunities to spent time with friends and other family members. Isolation and overwhelming commitment often leads to social and emotional withdrawal or depression in otherwise healthy adults. Others have reported high levels of symptoms of depression among the grandparent carers; for example Fuller-Thompson and colleagues (1997) reported that grandparent carers appeared to be at greater risk for elevated symptoms of depression than other elders (25% vs. 15%) and Burnette (2000) found elevated symptoms of depression among Latina grandparents caring for children with special needs. Our finding that 57% of grandparent carers reporting high (>16) symptom scores raises the concern that grandparents raising children with disabilities may be at further increased risk. These findings pose a challenge to researchers to further discern the impact of poverty, presence of disability, and other factors on the prevalence of symptoms of depression among grandparent carers. It also challenges workers to recognize such concerns among this population, and to develop and deliver more effective interventions.

Differences attributable to caregiving duration was another factor. We observed that there were a number of grandparents in our sample caring for adolescent or adult grandchildren. In one instance caregiving had lasted 35 years. This phenomenon raises several concerns, related mostly to the age of the grandparents and their longevity. If they continue to provide primary care for a child who then becomes an adult, their caregiving responsibilities may be of extended duration and will take them well into their own old age. Since most grandparents in the study were elderly to begin with, there were concerns about the ability of the grandparents to be alive and in good health as their grandchild grew into adolescence and beyond. However, these grandchildren often had multiple, life-long disabling conditions and caregiving needs will most likely continue into adulthood. This increases the likelihood that the grandparents will not be able to provide family type care for as long as it may be needed.

COMMENTARY

Given what we found, we see three particular concerns for child welfare and other workers who encounter grandparent carers of children with disabilities: the development of interventions, facilitating access to formal services, and planning for the future. To date, targeted interventions for caregiving grandparents have been limited, often because of a lack of funds. Intervention efforts have often focused on low cost options such as the development of support groups (see McCallion et al., 2000). It is also reported that the most stressed grandparents were unable to use such groups because of a lack of formal or informal respite services to care for children while they attend the group (Minkler et al., 1993). Workers must be advocates for the development of needed supports and must play roles in the design and delivery of successful and useful group and individual interventions for grandparents caring for children with disabilities. In addition, workers must also address the respite, transportation, and other resource barriers that prevent grandparents from using available services.

Our findings revealed that many grandparents experienced stress and uncertainty when attempting to secure help or specialty services related to the children's disabilities and needs. Indeed, grandparents reported themselves to be low users of existing services but in high need of services and benefits. This speaks to eligibility, access, knowledge, and other barriers with which workers may be of assistance in resolving. A particular concern is the grandparents' often undefined role with regard to guardianship and ability to speak for the natural, albeit absent, parent. This legally "grey" area begs for clarification as more skip-generation adults are facing long-term carer roles in our society. Without the ability to legally speak as a natural parent in matters of health care, education, and social services, and receive compensation or benefits from federal and state sources for their work as permanent carers, grandparents caring for children with special needs are significantly disadvantaged and placed in often untenable situations. Workers need to be cognizant of this concern and work toward helping grandparents clarify their legal status and authority in relation to their grandchildren and obtain public benefits as primary carers, free of discrimination.

REFERENCES

Barnhill, S. (1996). Three generations at risk: Imprisoned women, their children, and grandmother caregivers. *Generations, 20*(1), 39-40.
Biegel, D.E. and Blum, A. (Eds.) (1990). *Aging and caregiving: Theory, research, and policy.* Newbury Park, CA: Sage Publications, Inc.
Burnette, D. (1999). Social relationships of Latino grandparent caregivers: A role theory perspective. *The Gerontologist, 39*(1), 49-58.

Burnette, D. (1999). Custodial grandparents in Latino families: Patterns of service use and predictors of unmet needs. *Social Work, 44*(1), 22-34.

Burnette, D. (1997). Grandparents raising grandchildren in the inner city. *Families In Society, 78*(5), 489-501.

Burton, L. (1992). Black grandparents rearing children of drug addicted parents: Stressors, outcomes, and social services needs. *The Gerontologist, 32*(6), 744-751.

Cantor, M.H. (1991). Family and community: Changing roles in an aging society. *Gerontologist, 31*(3), 337-346.

Dubowitz, H., Feigelman, S., Harrington, D., Starr, R., and Zuravin, S. (1994). Children in kinship care: How do they fare? *Children and Youth Services Review, 16*(1-2), 85-106.

Flint, M. and Perez-Porter, M. (1997). Grandparent caregivers: Legal and economic issues. *Journal of Gerontological Social Work, 28*(1-2), 63-76.

Fuller-Thomson, E., Minkler, M. and Driver, D. (1997). A profile of grandparents raising grandchildren in the US. *The Gerontologist, 37*(3), 406-411.

Gibson, R.C. (1991). Race and the self-reported health of elderly persons. *Journals of Gerontology, 46*(5), S235-S242.

Gibson, R.C. (1991). Age-by-race differences in the health and functioning of elderly persons. *Journal of Aging and Health, 3*(3), 335-351.

Hanson, L. and Opsahl, I. (1996). Kinship caregiving: Law and policy. *Clearinghouse Review, 30*(5), 481-500.

Hays, R.D. and Stewart, A.L. (1990). The structure of self-reported health in chronic disease patients. *Psychological Assessment, 2*(1), 22-30.

Heller, T. and Factor, A. (1991). Permanency planning for adults with mental retardation living with family caregivers. *American Journal on Mental Retardation, 96*(2), 163-176.

Huyck, M.H. (1991). Predicates of personal control among middle-aged and young-old men and women in middle America. *International Journal of Aging and Human Development, 32*(4), 261-275.

Janicki, M., McCallion, P., Force, L.T., Bishop, K., and LePore, P. (1998). Area agency on aging outreach and assistance for households with older carers of an adult with a developmental disability. *Journal of Aging and Social Policy, 10*(1), 13-36.

Jendrek, M.P. (1994a). Grandparents who parent their grandchildren: Circumstances and decisions. *The Gerontologist, 34*(2), 206-216.

Jendrek, M.P. (1994b). Policy concerns of white grandparents who provide regular care for their grandchildren. *Journal of Gerontological Social Work, 23*(1-2), 175-200.

Karp, N. (1996). Legal problems of grandparents and other kinship caregivers. *Generations, 20*(1), 57-60.

Kelley, S.J., Yorker, B.C., and Whiteley, D. (1997). To grandma's house we go . . . and stay. *Journal of Gerontological Nursing,* 13-20.

Kramer, B.J. (1997). Differential predictors of strain and gain among husbands caring for wives with dementia. *The Gerontologist, 37*(2), 239-49.

Kraus, M.W. and Seltzer, M.M. (1993). Current well-being and future plans of older caregiving mothers. *Irish Journal of Psychology, 14*(1), 48-63.

Krauss, M.W. and Seltzer, M.M. (1993). Coping strategies among older mothers of adults with retardation: A life-span developmental perspective. In Turnbull, A.P., Patterson, J.M. et al. (Eds.) *Cognitive coping, families, and disability.* (pp. 173-182). Baltimore, MD: Paul H. Brookes Publishing.

Markides, K.S. and Miranda, M.R. (Eds.) (1997). *Minorities, aging, and health.* Thousand Oaks, CA: Sage Publications, Inc.

McCallion, P. and Toseland, R. (1993). Empowering families of adolescents and adults with developmental disabilities. *Families in Society, 74*(10), 579-587.

Minkler, M., Driver, D., Roe, K.M., and Bedeian, K. (1993). Community interventions to support grandparent caregivers. *The Gerontologist, 33*(6), 807-811.

Minkler, M., Fuller-Thomson, E., Miller, D., and Driver, D. (1997. Depression in grandparents raising grandchildren: Results of a national longitudinal study. *Archives of Family Medicine, 6*(5), 445-452.

Minkler, M., and Roe, K.M. (1993). *Grandmothers as caregivers: Raising children of the crack cocaine epidemic.* Newbury Park, CA: Sage Publications, Inc.

Minkler, M. Roe, K.M., and Price, M. (1992). The physical and emotional health of grandmothers raising grandchildren in the crack cocaine epidemic. *The Gerontologist, 32*(6), 752-761.

Mullen, F. (1996). Public benefits: Grandparents, grandchildren, and welfare reform. *Generations, 20*(1), 61-64.

Pruchno, R. (1995, September). *Grandparents in American Society: Review of recent literature.* Bethesda, MD: NIA

Nickens, H.W. (1995). The role of race/ethnicity and social class in minority health status. *Health Service Review, 30*(1-2), 151-162.

Pearlin, L.I. and Schooler, C. (1978). The structure of coping. *Journal of Health and Social Behavior, 19,* 2-21.

Pinson-Millburg, N.M., Schlossberg, N.K., and Pyle, M. (1996). Grandparents raising grandchildren. *Journal of Counseling and Development, 74*(6), 548-555.

Pruchno, R., Hicks-Patrick, J., and Burant, C. (1997). African American and white mothers of adults with chronic disabilities: Caregiving burden and satisfaction. *Family Relations, 46,* 335-346.

Radloff, L.S. (1977). The CES-D Scale: A self-report depression scale for research in the general population. *Applied Psychological Measurement, 1*(3), 385-401.

Scannapieco, M., Hegar, R.L., and McAlpine, C. (1997). Kinship care and foster care: A comparison of characteristics and outcomes. *Families in Society, 78*(5), 480-488.

Seltzer, M.M., Krauss, M.W., and Janicki, M.P. (Eds.) (1994). *Life course perspectives on adulthood and old age.* Washington, DC: American Association on Mental Retardation.

Seltzer, M.M., and Krauss, M.W. (1994). Aging parents with coresident adult children: The impact of lifelong caregiving. In M. Seltzer (Ed.); M. Krauss (Ed.); M. Janicki (Eds.). *Life course perspectives on adulthood and old age.* (pp. 3-18). Washington, DC: American Association on Mental Retardation.

Shore, R.J. and Hayslip, B. (1994). Custodial grandparenting. Implications for children's development. In Gottfried and Gottfried (Eds.), *Redefining families: Implications for children's development* (pp. 171-218). New York: Plenum Press.

Smith, P.K. (1991). Introduction: The study of grandparenthood. In P.K. Smith (Ed.), *The psychology of grandparenthood* (pp. 1-16). London: Routledge.

Smith, G.C., Fullmer, E.M., and Tobin, S. (1994). Living outside the system: An exploration of older families who do not use day programs. In M. Seltzer, M. Krauss, & M.P. Janicki (Ed.) *Life course perspectives on adulthood and old age.* (pp. 19-37). Washington, DC: American Association on Mental Retardation.

Stewart, A.L., Hays, R.D., and Ware, J.E. (1988). The MOS short-form general health survey: Reliability and validity in a patient population. *Medical Care*, *26*(7), 724-735.

Stump, T.E., Clark, D.O., Johnson, R.J., and Wolinsky, F.D. (1997). Structure of health status among Hispanic, African American, and white older adults. *Journals of Gerontology: Series B: Psychological and Social Sciences*, *52*B, 49-60.

Toseland, R.W., O'Donnell, J.C., Engelhardt, J.B., Richie, J., Jue, D., and Banks, S.M. (1997). Outpatient geriatric evaluation and management: Is there an investment effect? *The Gerontologist*, *37*(3), 324-332.

Grandparent Carers II:
Service Needs and Service Provision Issues

Philip McCallion, PhD, ACSW
Matthew P. Janicki, PhD
Lucinda Grant-Griffin, PhD
Stacey Kolomer, CSW

SUMMARY. A demonstration project was undertaken in two of New York City's five boroughs using an intervention model to assess how a three-prong approach using outreach, provision of support groups, and case management could be used to aid grandparents acting as primary carers for children with developmental delay or disabilities. Three small community-based agencies participated in the demonstration. Several common themes were identified that warrant attention when working with older adults who assume later-age parenting roles: (1) recruitment, (2) pressing grandparent problems, (3) unresponsive service systems, (4) falling between the cracks, (5) mutual support, and (6) need for long-term planning. *[Article copies available for a fee from The Haworth Document Delivery Service: 1-800-342-9678. E-mail address: <getinfo@haworthpressinc. com> Website: <http://www.HaworthPress.com>]*

Philip McCallion is Assistant Professor and Hartford Geriatric Social Work Faculty Scholar, and Matthew P. Janicki is Research Professor, School of Social Welfare, University at Albany. Lucinda Grant-Griffin is Policy Analyst, New York State Office of Mental Retardation and Developmental Disabilities, Albany, NY. Stacey Kolomer is a Doctoral Candidate associated with the Centre on Intellectual Disabilities, School of Social Welfare, University at Albany.

Address correspondence to: Philip McCallion, PhD, RI 208, University at Albany, 135 Western Avenue, Albany, NY 12222 (E-mail: mcclion@csc.albany.edu).

Funding for this project was provided by the Joseph P. Kennedy, Jr., Foundation.

[Haworth co-indexing entry note]: "Grandparent Carers II: Service Needs and Service Provision Issues." McCallion, Philip et al. Co-published simultaneously in *Journal of Gerontological Social Work* (The Haworth Press, Inc.) Vol. 33, No. 3, 2000, pp. 57-84; and: *Grandparents as Carers of Children with Disabilities: Facing the Challenges* (ed: Philip McCallion and Matthew Janicki) The Haworth Press, Inc., 2000, pp. 57-84. Single or multiple copies of this article are available for a fee from The Haworth Document Delivery Service [1-800-342-9678, 9:00 a.m. - 5:00 p.m. (EST). E-mail address: getinfo@haworthpressinc. com].

KEYWORDS. Service needs of grandparent carers, support groups for carers, problems and stressors of grandparent carers, unresponsive service systems

Older adults living in low income, urban neighborhoods are increasingly assuming caregiving responsibilities for grandchildren when such care is needed, but may be doing so with the few resources at their disposal. Such assumption of care responsibilities has been associated with poverty, crack cocaine usage, alcohol abuse, AIDS, child abuse and neglect, incarceration, immaturity and violence interfering with the biological parent's ability to care for his or her children (Barnhill, 1996; Burton, 1992; Minkler, Roe, & Price, 1992). In this regard, the burgeoning literature on skip-generation or grandparent caregiving suggests that grandparent carers experience much stress (Burton, 1992; Fuller-Thompson, Minkler, & Driver, 1997), are often reluctant to accept needed services because they feel judged by others, including their caseworkers (Crumbley & Little, 1997), have health concerns and cumulative life experience difficulties prior to the assumption of this responsibility (Minkler et al., 1992; Strawbridge, Wallhagen, Shema, & Kaplan, 1997), and over-report their own well-being and deny their own needs, lest such admissions be used to justify removing the children (Jendrek, 1994). There are also indications that because such assumptive carer situations are overly concentrated in urban, low income areas, there are likely to be more social and environmental stressors (such as, poverty, violence, and substance abuse) and fewer supportive resources (such as, informal support networks, and school and human service agency assistance) (Fuller-Thompson et al., 1997; Harden, Clark, & Maguire, 1997; Venkatesh, 1997). Consideration of the service needs of grandparent carers must therefore begin with a recognition that grandparents and the children they care for experience multiple problems, and needs often go unmet in economically depressed communities lacking in public and private resources to address those needs.

Measures are required to address the service needs of all caregiving grandparents. However, this report is particularly concerned about grandparent-headed households that include at least one child with a developmental disability. Despite the fact that many of the already listed causes of grandparent assumption of care have long been known to also have strong linkages to causes of intellectual and other developmental disabilities, and that care of a child with a developmental disability may further increase grandparent isolation and need for support, there has been little consideration in the existing literature of grandparents caring for children with developmental disabilities. Children with developmental disabilities cared for by grandparents represent a group who is fortunate to have caring family members willing to accept this responsibility late in their own lives. However, they also represent a particularly needy group. Legal status concerns for all caregiving grandparents are often magnified when the child has a developmental disability; for example, physicians in emergency rooms are less likely to be willing to provide services without a signed legal guardian consent (Personal communication, Perez-Porter, March 1998). In addition, children with developmental disabilities, despite the best efforts of their carers, often are unable to access needed services, particularly educational services. Finally, children with developmental disabilities from multi-cultural households have traditionally been under-represented on the service rolls of formal agencies, and are asked to fit into existing services patterns rather than have their unique, individual needs addressed in a culturally sensitive manner (McCallion, Janicki, & Grant-Griffin, 1997). This situation is likely to be even more prevalent in grandparent carer situations.

The presence of a grandchild with a developmental disability, therefore, is likely to add to the stresses experienced by grandparent carers. However, the development of service models requires greater understanding of why existing services are not sufficient. Some of the issues to be considered are (1) lack of an institutional host for grandparent services; (2) lack of sensitivity in service provision; and (3) lack of providers willing to shape services to grandparent needs.

LACK OF AN INSTITUTIONAL HOST

Interventions targeted at grandparents have been limited, often because of a lack of funds. Grandparents also fall between the cracks of agency responsibility. It is unresolved as to whether services should be provided and coordinated through aging agencies or foster care agencies, where needs of informal grandparent carers fit in, and what is the appropriate involvement of schools and disability services agencies when special education and disability-related needs exist. A recent analysis of calls received by the New York City Department for the Aging's Grandparent Resource Center illustrates the extent of grandparent problems, and the many agency services they intersect. During the first nine months of operation, the Center received calls from approximately 800 grandparents, 75% of whom reported caring for a child presenting with, or at risk for, a developmental delay or disability. Information gleaned from the Resource Center's hotline (Personal communication, Pyle, 1997) suggested that grandparent carer problems fall into five principal areas:

1. *Financial* (grandparents have difficulty accessing public assistance, emergency cash, and Medicaid).
2. *Guardianship* (informal transfers of responsibility for caregiving for the child with a disability usually mean that legal guardianship has not

been established, posing difficulties when permissions for medical care and other services are needed).

3. *Respite* (grandparents have no time off from caregiving).

4. *Emotional support* (some grandparent carers have not resolved their feelings about the death, drug addiction or absence of their own child [the grandchild's parent]; others may not feel supported by their spouse and other family members, feel isolated, and fear for the future).

5. *Problems with service systems* (grandparents have difficulty negotiating the maze of social services, child welfare, disability, education, housing, medical, and aging services).

The absence of an institutional location and priority for these service needs has meant few resources for grandparent care. Service development efforts to date have focused on low cost options such as establishing support groups. Grandparents do report both a need for such groups and increased satisfaction and coping from their use (Minkler, Driver, Roe, & Bedeian, 1993). This has led to efforts to expand their availability. For example, the Brookdale Foundation in New York has supported the development of support group models, and has funded their dissemination throughout the United States. However, few groups have been developed so far in low income communities, and it is also reported that many grandparents are unable to use such groups because of a lack of respite services to care for children while they attend the group (Minkler et al., 1993).

LACK OF SENSITIVITY IN SERVICE PROVISION

Sensitivity concerns fall into two areas: (1) cultural sensitivity, and (2) grandparenting sensitivity.

Cultural sensitivity. There are indications that persons from minority cultures are generally less likely to participate in service programs because they face economic, religious, transportation and insurance barriers to participation, they do not feel welcomed in the locations where the interventions are offered, or the interventions are simply not designed to meet their needs (McCallion, Janicki, & Grant-Griffin, 1997; Henderson, Gutierrez-Mayka, Garcia, & Boyd, 1993). However, where concerted efforts have been made to develop interventions for persons from minority cultures, participants have been located and have reported benefits from participation (see for example Henderson et al., 1993, Minkler, Driver, Roe, & Bedian, 1993).

Investigations of low usage of formal interventions by family carers from minority sub-populations have noted greater availability of extended family supports, suspicion of formal structures, and cultural beliefs that one should take care of one's own (Lockery, 1991; Sung, 1995; Sakauye, 1989). For example, despite the stresses and financial strains, many grandparents report that caring for their grandchildren is simply part of their role as grandparents, and that no sacrifice is too great to maintain their grandchildren within the family (Burton, 1992). One's culture (i.e., the values, beliefs, customs, behaviors, structures, and identity by which a group of people define themselves–Axelson, 1993) does appear to be an important influence on one's willingness to use services. However, assuming that identification with a particular culture means strict adherence to a specific set of beliefs and practices may inadvertently stereotype minority families from the same cultural group (Gratton & Wilson, 1988). Also, the experience of historic discrimination for all, legal status concerns for some, and the foreignness of services which have been developed *for,* rather than *by* the communities to be served may be more important reasons for why families from minority cultures choose not to use formal services (McCallion et al., 1997). For grandparents assuming carer roles, low levels of actual use of community supports do not necessarily mean that more formal assistance is not needed; conversely, it may mean that they may find offered services inappropriate to their needs.

Grandparenting sensitivity. As noted by Kolomer (2000), grandparent carers may not seek services because they feel that care of kin is the responsibility of families and should not require subsidy or support, or they may feel ashamed or judged because they have assumed care in situations where their own child has failed to adequately care for the grandchild. Those older adults caring for children with a developmental delay or disability may also share the concerns of other older carers that to acknowledge need may result in the removal and institutionalization (or foster placement) of the child (McCallion & Tobin, 1993). Equally, they may be unaware of the ways in which services have changed from when they first parented, and the range and nature of services currently available. Put simply, they are unlikely to seek services about which they do not know. Eligibility requirements, waiting periods and other rules that service agencies require compound this problem (Kolomer, 2000). A lack of connectedness to services and service providers may be the most critical issue here.

LACK OF PROVIDERS WILLING TO SHAPE SERVICES TO GRANDPARENT NEEDS

Venkatesh (1997) has suggested that service agencies serving urban, low income communities fall into three classes or tiers. The first, or the elite tier, are those agencies that are well established, influence how resources are distributed in the community, and have survived over the years in the face of changing circumstances. They have a stable base of resources, serve established client groups and usually have a sizeable staff, clear procedures for services and the respect of funding mechanisms and sources. When new service needs are recognized, this is the group of agencies to whom tradition-al funders (such as governments and foundations) are most likely to turn to. However, Venkatesh (1997) notes that the hard earned stability of these agencies also causes them to concentrate on what they know and to draw upon existing programs, workers and procedures to meet new needs–but not in ways that may potentially take resources from established client groups. The absence of a defined funding stream and the lack of an institutional host at the state level for grandparent carer services can deter such agencies from committing resources to these families.

The second group, mid-tier agencies, is made up of generally smaller, less well-established agencies that offer only a modest set of programs and ser-vices. However, these agencies are more likely to reach out to neglected sectors of the community, such as grandparent carers. Often their very devel-opment may have been the result of identification of such unmet needs, generally from the personal experiences of the organization's leaders or di-rect interactions with potential consumers of services. These are not well-re-sourced organizations, and usually meet needs identified by their communi-ties by shifting staff, programs, and resources. From a funder perspective, they do not have the stability and track record of the elite level organizations and are often not the first choice for the funding of new initiatives.

The third tier is composed of grassroots providers, often individuals or social groups. They may also be non-providers, such as social/fraternal orga-nizations that voluntarily assume a provider role using their own resources. In impoverished communities these providers often serve the most isolated (i.e., those who lack knowledge of services, prefer informality to appoint-ments, forms and formal means of interaction, feel victimized or controlled when they accept services, and who may even in the past have had antagonis-tic relationships with more formal organizations). Many grandparent carers fall into this category of consumers. Despite serving the most needy, such providers rarely receive resources from funders, because they are not known, and do not have professional staff, a conventional history of providing formal services, a "funding record," or even the means to receive and account for monies.

There have been some efforts by existing elite agencies to reach out to grandparenting families, but with mixed results. Using staff (usually para-professionals) drawn from grandparents' own communities, outreach to churches and civic groups, and public service announcements, these first tier agencies have attempted to draw grandparent-lead families into their existing programs, and to establish satellite offices in their communities. An assump-tion in these approaches, as yet unproven, is that everyone can be fitted into existing program and service models (McCallion et al., 1997). Yet, the services offered by these agencies have been limited by the availability of grants and other specific funding, and efforts have tended to be short-lived. As a consequence, grandparents and their needs have not been integrated into the supports of existing funding streams and programs (Personal communication, Pyle, March 1998). Such approaches also have generally failed to recognize the strengths offered by locally based mid- and third tier "multi-cultural agencies" (i.e., agencies targeting a particular minority cultural group), or to involve them in the expansion of services to under-served populations.

Mid- and third-tier agencies have not been part of the traditional services network because meeting the needs of families from diverse cultures has not been a funding or policy priority, underfunding has meant that multi-cultural agencies have had difficulty supporting the professional staff expected by funders and regulators, elite tier agency administrators have resisted sharing resources, and service systems have only recently switched from personal responsibility perspectives which multi-cultural agencies did not share, to emphasizing empowerment approaches which they do (Iglehart & Becerra, 1996; McCallion & Grant-Griffin, in press; Venkatesh, 1997). Yet, ironically, these agencies have always existed in one form or another. Some are church based, and others are fraternal in nature. Many offer a combination of social, cultural and human services. Most of their funding is raised within the community they serve. They serve locally based cultural communities which traditionally have not been offered services, where existing services are not appropriate, or where a cultural community's language and customs make accessing formal services difficult. They are also:

1. easily accessed because they are close by to those persons they serve, do not require appointments, and have longer hours of operation than other agencies;
2. seen by families as more nurturing, supportive and likely to understand cultural concerns;
3. more likely to see culture as an intervention facilitator rather than an intervention barrier; and
4. based upon empowerment approaches, are oriented toward helping families to change their environment, rather than looking at families for the source of the presenting problems.

Given the lack of identifiable examples of such mid- and third tier agencies being drawn into specifically serving grandparent carers with children at home with identified or suspected developmental delay or disabilities, the lack of a demonstrable model for supports of such carers, and the lack of a public agency institutional host and funder targeting such grandparent carers, it was decided to undertake a demonstration project with three primary objectives: (1) the assessment of grandparents in such carer roles and their primary support needs, (2) identification and testing of a model of supports that could involve agencies close to their constituents, and (3) the development of interest for an institutional host and funder. Janicki, McCallion, Kolomer, and Grant-Griffin (2000) have reported on the first of these objectives and Kolomer (2000) has noted some of the features of the second objective. This report covers primarily the latter two objectives.

THE PROJECT

In 1997, the senior authors approached the Joseph P. Kennedy, Jr. Foundation and requested funding for a demonstration project that would address the three objectives noted above. The project was thus designed to be the first effort to systematically examine the needs of grandparents caring for children with intellectual and other developmental disabilities, and to identify and field test a service model to assist them. Core aspects of this model included the use of mid-tier multi-cultural agencies, the provision of intensive case management services, the offering of support groups, and interaction and advocacy with local and state aging and developmental disabilities oversight agencies to ensure continuation of supports after the completion of the grant period.

Funding for the Grandparent Assistance Demonstration Project was received from the Joseph P. Kennedy, Jr., Foundation in Washington, DC. The project ran from 1997 to 1999 and involved a 12-month service demonstration period carried out in several low income neighborhoods of New York City's boroughs of Bronx and Queens. The project began with a competitive bid period designed to identify three agencies willing to participate. To identify the three agencies, bid packages were sent to approximately 100 not-for-profit disability and social service agencies of varying size, known to the state's developmental disabilities services agency or to New York City's area agency on aging. Eligibility was restricted to legally established not-for-profit agencies which provide the majority of their services in either of two targeted boroughs, whose programs serve persons from various minority groups, and which could demonstrate capacity or prior experience in working with grandparent carers. Several bidder conferences were held to ensure that interested agencies understood the project's requirements and would demonstrate, in their proposals, due diligence, innovation and a genuine commitment to the project. Three agencies were selected from among the eight proposals received by the due date. Selection was made by a review panel (consisting of representatives from state and local aging and developmental disabilities agencies, advocates for grandparent carers and a grandparent carer) which rated received proposals against pre-set criteria drawn from the request for proposals.

THE PROJECT MODEL

The intervention model used by the Grandparent Assistance Demonstration Project was composed of a three-prong approach to providing support and assistance. The first was a component that involved *aggressive outreach* to recruit grandparent participants; the second was the use of grandparent-oriented *mutual support groups* initially developed and tested by the New York City Department for the Aging and specially tailored (by project staff) for grandparents providing primary care for children/adults with a developmental disability; and the third was a course of *intensive case management* and personal counseling designed to aid problem solving. From the grandparent participant perspective the model required the grandparents to agree to confer with outreach workers, attend support meetings, and work with the agency's caseworker to help solve identified service eligibility, entitlement, or access problems. Oversight and process controls were provided and administered by the senior authors, as the project's principal investigators.

THE AGENCIES

Agency One was a small agency located in the borough of Queens, founded by the parents of a child with a developmental disability. Although the staff was largely Latino, the needs for service in the local community were such that they provide parent training, case management, respite, and some day services to African, Caribbean, African-American, Haitian, as well as Latino families. In 1996 they were approached by a number of grandparent carers in need, and without any formal resources began offering services to them.

Agency Two was primarily an African-American agency located in the borough of Queens. Family established, this growing not-for-profit agency had at its core transportation services both for elderly and frail persons and special education students. Experiencing growing stability, the agency had recently expanded into case management, respite, recreation and some residential and day services. Staff were also serving families of varied ethnic backgrounds. Using their transportation program they were also coming into increasing contact with grandparent carers, and found themselves providing additional services to such families, without any formal funding.

Agency Three was located in the borough of The Bronx and was primarily a residential provider to persons with AIDS as well as to persons with developmental disabilities. The agency mission was to provide care to those who have been denied compassionate treatment because of race, gender, sexual orientation, health, developmental level, criminal, or substance abuse history. Staff were aware of the concerns of grandparent carers, some of whom were caring for the children of their residential services clients. They were also concerned about the grandparent carers they came in contact with in the neighborhoods in which their programs were located.

Agencies One and Two were mid-tier agencies. Agency Three was considered as approaching elite tier status because of its size, level of staffing, and more formal program structures. However, its continued orientation to vulnerable and marginalized populations, and its willingness to commit its own resources and reorient programs to serve grandparents, showed that it still possessed mid-tier characteristics.

THE DEMONSTRATION

Agency preparations. The participating agencies were expected to designate a project director, grandparent program case manager, and support group facilitator, recruit a minimum of 30 grandparents each caring for at least one grandchild with a developmental disability, complete a comprehensive assessment of each family's needs, offer intensive case management and support group services, follow the families for 12 months, and to seek continuation funding to aid those families who continued to need them. The staff designated to participate in the project were required to attend a two-day training institute organized by the project leaders and to attend bimonthly project cluster meetings. The agenda for the training institute is shown in Figure 1.

The institute exposed participants to the varying agencies, regulations and service needs that had been identified as most crucial to improving supports and removing service barriers for caregiving grandparents. State and local agency representatives, grandparent advocates and grandparent carers themselves comprised the institute's faculty. Emphasis was placed on providing the participants with the critical information and personal contacts that would enable them to effectively negotiate their way through the different agencies, resolve eligibility disputes, and locate alternative services where they encountered barriers. During the institute it became apparent that staff from the participating agencies were already quite skilled and possessed knowledge in these areas and so the sessions became more interactive than didactic as each shared their knowledge. This became the *modus operandi* during the bimonthly meetings over the 12 months of the project. During these meetings, participants shared strategies that worked for particular grandparent service

FIGURE 1. Agenda for Agency Training

DAY ONE

Overview of Grandparent Assistance Project

Overview of the State Developmental Disabilities Services Agency and Introduction of Borough Liaisons

Overview of New York City Department of Mental Health, Mental Retardation and Alcoholism Services

New York State Adoption Demonstration Project

Grandparent Carer Issues

How to Run Effective Support Group Meetings

Kinship Foster Care–Issues and Services

DAY TWO

Benefits, Guardianship, Eligibility, Proxies and Other Legal Issues

The Special Education Process and Guardian's Rights

Helping Grandparents to Take Care of Themselves

Resources and Benefits for Children with Developmental Disabilities

needs, supported each other's efforts on particularly difficult cases, and identified areas where they and the project leaders might jointly approach funding and regulatory agencies seeking to educate them about the needs of grandparents.

Support groups. The primary intervention for the project was support groups. Each agency was required to identify an individual to lead their grandparent support groups (oversight was provided by the designated project person). Groups of 8-10 grandparents were offered a minimum of six support group meetings (mostly held fortnightly). To facilitate attendance, agencies offered in-home or on-site respite and assistance with transportation. Group leaders were trained using the project's support group training manual (see Figure 2), the contents of which were developed in response to the recommendations of focus groups of grandparents and grandparent advocates. The manual also made extensive use of existing proven grandparent support materials (see for example, Grandparent Resource Center, 1998a, 1998b; Samuel Sadin Institute on Law, 1997a, 1997b, 1998). The premise for the support group intervention contents was the recognition that grandparent caregiving needs varied widely, the children being cared for were of all ages, and disability-related needs required educational as well as support components for the group.

Support group leaders were encouraged to work with each group of 8-10 grandparents to identify the six sections of the manual they would be most

FIGURE 2. Support Group Meeting Topics

1. Developmental Delays and Disabilities
2. Getting Services
3. Your Grandchild's Education
4. The Teen Years
5. State DD Agency Services
6. Skills for Caring
7. Problems Behaviors
8. Helping a Child with a Disability
9. Custody and Guardianship
10. Your Grandchild's Parents
11. Planning for the Future

Each session also included a segment on "Taking Care of the Carer"

interested in having presented in their sessions. Topics not only included items that the grandparents chose which addressed their grandchildren's needs, but also items that would help the grandparent take care of themselves (including stress reduction, relaxation, nutrition, and taking care of one's own health needs).

Case management. The agencies were also required to provide case management related to the problems raised by the participating grandparents. Each agency designated a staff person responsible for case management and counseling. The project's initial orientation provided information on cross-cutting resources and other issues that grandparents may face. However, it was noted that the agencies had casework structures that were already responding to the diverse needs of low income carers (e.g., help with housing, interventions with social and health agencies, benefits counseling, etc.).

FINDINGS

Data Collection

Agencies were supplied with a common intake questionnaire, which was to be completed for each participating grandparent. The intake questionnaire was a 210-item protocol designed to gather demographic, health and mental health information on the grandparent carers, as well as demographics, legal status and disability diagnoses on the children. The protocol also gathered information on formal service use and needs, and appraisals of the grandparent's relationship with the grandchild's parents. A Spanish language version was provided for use with those grandparents who were Spanish speaking. A backward and forward translation process was used. Two bilingual translators helped in preparing the Spanish version; one translator was a community leader working with grandparents who also ensured that the translations of the measures were culturally and linguistically appropriate (Zambrana, 1991).

Minutes were kept of all project meetings and a semi-structured debriefing interview was conducted with each of the three participating agencies (see Figure 3). On a post-hoc basis, the minutes and the transcripts of the semi-structured interviews were reviewed for common themes to understand significant milestones and processes of the project.

Grandparent and Child Intake Findings

The three agencies recruited 120 grandparent carers where at least one of the children being cared for had a developmental delay or disability. Intake questionnaires were completed on 97. Six of the grandparents "disappeared" before data could be collected. Their loss was attributed to being in jeopardy because of legal status or indebtedness or eviction concerns (indeed, it appears that such concerns resulted in their abrupt relocations out of the area). The remainder of the non-responders were individuals who were interested in receiving help, but who were not willing either to attend support groups or to complete questionnaires. A majority of these were Latino carers. Selected information about the 97 grandparent carers for whom intake questionnaires were completed and the children they cared for is found in Tables 1 and 2.

Table 1 shows that the majority of grandparent carers were female (94%) with an average age of 60 (*s.d.* = 10 years; range: 40-82). Some 79% were African-Americans, 36% had an available spouse, 25% were educated beyond high school, and 31% were also holding a job. They cared for at least one grandchild for an average of seven years. Most grandparents were caring for one or two grandchildren, but some were caring for as many as seven. Most of the grandparents were low users of any formal services (such as, case management, assistance with housing issues and support groups), using on the average only one of these services. When asked about what services they needed, they reported needing at least five additional different formal services.

Of the grandchildren, 171 were being cared for by the 97 grandparent carers. Table 2 shows that 57% of the children were male with an average age of 11 years (*s.d.* = 4.9; range: 2-25). Eight children were over 20 and represented long term caregiving by grandparents. Although many grandparents reported that they had legal responsibility for their grandchildren (75%),

FIGURE 3. Grandparent Assistance Demonstration Project

Semi-Structured Debriefing Questions.

1. *Give an overview of your agency's experience of participating in this project:*
   - what did you expect to happen?
   - what turned out as you expected?
   - what turned out differently than you expected?

2. *When you started the project, what was your plan for recruitment?*
   - what worked?
   - what didn't work?
   - what changes in the plan did you implement?
   - how well did those changes work?
   - what recommendations would you make to another agency beginning to recruit grandparents?

3. *At the beginning of the project we provided you with a lot of materials regarding services that grandparents might use:*
   - which materials did you find most useful?
   - which materials did you not find useful?
   - what other materials would have been helpful?

4. *Two days of training on services and service needs were provided at the beginning of the project:*
   - how helpful was this training?
   - what other types of training would have been helpful?

5. *You received a support group manual:*
   - how helpful were the materials in the manual?
   - have you used other materials during the meetings besides those in the manual?
   - would you recommend the development of any additional materials to be included in the manual?

6. *When you started the project, what was your plan for running the support groups?*
   - what worked?
   - what didn't work?
   - what changes in the plan did you implement?
   - how well did those changes work?
   - what recommendations would you make to another agency beginning support groups for grandparents?

7. *When you started the project, what was your plan for providing transportation to the support groups?*
   - what worked?
   - what didn't work?
   - what changes in the plan did you implement?
   - how well did those changes work?
   - what recommendations would you make to another agency beginning support groups for grandparents?

8. *When you started the project, what was your plan for providing respite so that grandparents could attend the support groups?*
   – what worked?
   – what didn't work?
   – what changes in the plan did you implement and how well did those changes work?
   – what recommendations would you make to another agency beginning support groups for grandparents?

9. *When you started the project, what was your plan for providing case management and other services assistance?*
   – what worked?
   – what didn't work?
   – what changes in the plan did you implement and how well did those changes work?
   – what recommendations would you make to another agency beginning to provide case management and other services assistance for grandparents?

10. *Describe the typical grandparent carer you have worked with?*

11. *Describe the most unusual grandparent carer situation you have worked with?*

12. *Describe the most difficult grandparent carer situation you have worked with?*

13. *In general, what are the most pressing service needs you encountered among grandparent carers?*

14. *Which service needs were the easiest to resolve?*
   – give an example and describe the steps you took.

15. *Which service needs were the most difficult to resolve?*
   – give an example and describe the steps you took.

16. *Describe your contacts with the following agencies on behalf of grandparents:*
   – indicate how helpful or unhelpful they were.
   – give examples of where you were able to get the services grandparents needed and where you were not.
   – describe problems in the rules and procedures in these agencies that prevent grandparents getting the services they need.
   - A. the local developmental disabilities services office
   - B. the Medicaid office
   - C. the Medicare office
   - D. ACS–foster care
   - E. Public Housing
   - F. Social Security
   - G. Hospitals and Clinics
   - H. Other Health Care Providers
   - I. Transportation Providers
   - J. Local Schools
   - K. Courts

17. *What are the skills you believe a worker needs to work effectively with these families?*

18. *How do you plan to continue providing services to the grandparent families you have identified?*

TABLE 1. Grandparent Demographics (n = 97)

Variable	%
Gender	
Female	94
Male	6
Age	
< 60	50
60-74	28
75+	12
Ethnicity	
African American	79
European	6
Hispanic/Latino	12
Native American	2
Other	1
Religion	
Catholic	15
Protestant	85
Marital Status	
Married/Live-in relationship	36
Divorced/Separated	24
Never Married	11
Widowed	29
Education	
Some High School	43
High School Graduate	32
Some College	19
College Graduate	6
Housing Situation	
Rent	55
Own	45
Employment Status	
Working	31

TABLE 2. Grandchild Demographics (n = 171)

Variable	%
Gender	
Female	43
Male	57
Age	
< 5	8
5-9	35
10-14	37
15-19	12
20+	8
Diagnoses given to grandparents	
Autism	9
Intellectual disability	26
Developmental disabilities	47
Cerebral palsy	3
Epilepsy	3
Attention deficit hyperactivity disorder	32
Neurologically impaired	14
Vision or hearing impaired	18
Learning problems	55
Speech problems	54
Multiple problems	55
Grandparent description of children's problems	
Behaviors that are difficult to control	63
Problems hearing and/or seeing	22
Health problems	43
Problems walking	17
Problems holding things	16
Other people having more than expected difficulty understanding child	41
Problems in school	52
Child not able to do things children of same age can do	53
Child has problems learning new things	53
Child is in special education class	71
Child is involved with guidance counselor and/or resource room	64

TABLE 2. (continued)

Legal status of child	
Kinship foster care	8
Grandparent, temporary court custody	11
Grandparent, court appointed guardian	41
Legally adopted by grandparent	12
Being established	4
Informal care	24
Legal responsibility of child	
Parent	20
Grandparent	75
Other	5

actual legal status included legal adoption (12%), kinship foster care (8%), ongoing court involvement in establishing status (56%), and informal care (24%).

Multiple problems or disabilities were identified for 55% of the sample, intellectual and other developmental disabilities were noted for 73%, and learning problems and attention deficit and hyperactivity disorders were a diagnosis for 55% and 32% respectively. Grandparents were also asked to indicate if a number of behaviors were present for their grandchildren as a way of identifying delays and disabilities not yet receiving formal diagnosis. Here, 71% of children were reported as being in a special education class, 52% reported problems in school, 63% had behaviors that were difficult to control, and 53% stated that their grandchild was not able to do things that other children of their age were able to do.

Agency Findings

All of the participating agencies commented on how gratifying it was to work with grandparent carers. One support group leader, herself a young mother, talked about how much she had learned from the grandparents, how concerned and committed they were to their grandchildren and positive their attitudes despite the hardships being endured. There were many challenging situations, as illustrated in the following vignette:

> Mrs. N. is a 77-year-old grandmother who raised her emotionally disturbed granddaughter and is now raising that granddaughter's three children, one of whom has been classified as multiply disabled. Mrs. N.

has never pursued establishing legal guardianship or benefits for her great grandchildren, and is struggling to maintain the family and her apartment on her own social security payments. Her health is compromised due to arthritis and several knee surgeries. Mrs. N. feels trapped because she and her great grandchildren are living in a second floor apartment waiting for a more accessible apartment to become available. However, she's not sure that she can afford what a new apartment would cost, and she is afraid that her landlord will evict her if he finds out that she is looking for alternative accommodations.

A number of common themes emerged from the review of minutes and the semi-structured interviews; these fell into the following areas: (1) recruitment, (2) pressing grandparent problems, (3) unresponsive service systems, (4) falling between the cracks, (5) mutual support, and (6) need for long-term planning.

Recruitment. All three agencies used a variety of means to recruit grandparent families. These included placing advertisements in local and ethnic newspapers, posting flyers in other agencies, churches, laundromats, bodegas, clinics, schools and senior centers, and identifying grandparent headed families among consumers of the agency's other programs. However, word of mouth was universally the most effective means of recruiting participants. One agency experienced success in recruiting teachers in a local school to talk about the program with the grandparents of their students. Staff at another agency talked with members of their local church, and all three agencies talked about the success of grandparents recruiting other grandparents.

Grandparents were reported to be generally suspicious of efforts to recruit them; they did not believe that the services promised would be offered. They were services-exhausted ("I need a case manager for all my case managers"), or they suspected that this was a pretext to remove the child. Trust was difficult to build, but not impossible. For example, one grandfather caring for a daughter and a granddaughter with a developmental disability joined the program because the executive director of one of the agencies was a member of his church, and he felt he could trust her not to try to take the children away.

Pressing grandparent problems. Grandparents were described as nice, loving, talkative, alone, stressed, overwhelmed, scared, needing reassurance, uncertain about how service systems worked, easily put off by denials of services and benefits–yet grateful for the assistance they received, and happy that they were preserving a home for their grandchildren. Some situations, however, required intervention on multiple levels:

Mrs. Q was 52 years old and caring for two grandchildren one of whom was multiply disabled and prone to explosive violent outbursts which necessitated 24 hour supervision. Mrs. Q was also caring for a sick and paralyzed spouse and had opened her home to six adult nephews and nieces, none of whom helped with caregiving or contributed to the household. Mortgage payments and utility bills were past due by many months and eviction was threatened. Her own health was deteriorating and agency staff suspected she was being physically abused by her grandson.

Each agency had several similar cases that required daily intervention. Specific services which agency staff obtained for grandparents that they had not or were unable to obtain for themselves can be found in Table 3.

TABLE 3. Agency Provided Services Used

	Grandparents (n = 97)	Grandchildren with DD (n = 174)
Speech/Physical/Occupational Therapy	22	
Residential		3
Housing	11	
Parenting Skills Training	38	
Connections to Other Human Services Agencies	21	
Health Care	41	6
Benefits–Medicaid/Food Stamps/ Social Security/Public Assistance	28	21
Establishing Eligibility for Developmental Disabilities Services		30
Respite	36	
Telephone Reassurance	62	
Budgeting Assistance	12	
Nutrition Assistance	44	
Home Modification	11	
Transportation	23	28
Summer Camp		45
Support Group	88	

Support groups, telephone reassurance, and case management were provided by the agencies. To the extent they were able (and usually when they were not able to get other agencies to provide these), the agencies also provided respite services and parent training. They found that providing transportation was often the key to enabling grandparents to access needed speciality services for the grandchild with a developmental disability. Particularly notable was what the agencies did in locating summer camps. Many grandparents were concerned about the welfare and safety of their grandchildren, and their own ability to cope during the summer months when school was out. Finding summer camps usually involved obtaining scholarships and other financial assistance so that grandchildren might attend. Despite several successes, agency staff generally reported great difficulty in locating suitable camps, and in finding the financial assistance that made attendance possible. Also, at least in New York City, the camps most likely to meet the needs of children with a developmental disability are usually completely booked by February. Without agency assistance, most grandparents anxious to access a summer camp for their grandchild would not have obtained, completed and returned the necessary paperwork on time.

Another important category of assistance was establishing eligibility for developmental disabilities services. Due to the informal nature of some caregiving situations and a lack of information in others, there were a number of children who were clearly eligible who had not been deemed so, and who, therefore, were not receiving services to which they might be entitled. For approximately thirty children the agencies reported playing a critical role in locating the necessary documentation, arranging for evaluations and advocating with the local developmental disabilities services office to have these children declared eligible. Again, this was a time-consuming process, with many potential barriers that required active participation of agency staff to ensure a successful outcome.

Unresponsive service systems. Many grandparents were found to have been denied benefits such as social security-disability and Medicaid to which they or their grandchildren were entitled, or to have given up on applying because of the need to travel to agency offices, wait for extended periods or provide documentation to which they did not have access. A principal intervention reported by all three agencies was to encourage grandparents to pursue these benefits either for the first time or to appeal previous denials. The latter proved to be a time-consuming process for agency staff, as they often had to accompany grandparents to these appeals, and, in approximately 25 cases, reported having to involve legal aid attorneys in the process before they obtained the benefit.

A majority of the participating grandparents lived in rented housing. Among those who owned their own homes, many lived in homes that were too small for the number of children now living there. Renter or homeowner, many grandparents were also concerned about the safety of their grandchildren and wished to move. In eleven instances, agencies reported that were able to find alternative and better housing for the families. However, they reported at least 20 other instances that they were unable to resolve (e.g., where homes were too small, landlords unresponsive, environments unsafe, and upper story apartments inaccessible for persons with disabilities). A critical concern identified was that existing subsidized and specialized housing projects were unwilling to accept grandparents with children, saying that they served only elderly adults or persons with disabilities.

The grandparents and their agency advocates experienced a great deal of frustration in trying to obtain special education services and ancillary supports through the schools. They also experienced difficulties in maintaining health services for both grandparent and grandchild as managed care companies dropped and added providers, dropped and added coverage, and hospitals and clinics placed limits on Medicaid recipients. The agencies were often overwhelmed trying to help grandparents maintain existing health services, and negotiate their way through the myriad paperwork systems.

Falling through the cracks. Many of the service and eligibility problems faced by the agencies resulted from grandparents "not fitting in." Staff reported that eligibility requirements assumed traditional family and guardianship situations, and required paperwork that often only parents would have access to. As one situation illustrates:

> They took Mrs. G.'s grandson away from her daughter in the middle of the night and dropped him off with Mrs. G. All he had was the clothing he was wearing. It was an abuse case. The child protective worker made her all kinds of promises about the help she would receive. Mrs. G. says that she didn't see any of that help. When she wouldn't agree to help terminate her daughter's parental rights and become a kinship foster care provider, but wanted to keep her grandson, they told her she was on her own. After a while Mrs. G. saw that she needed help in establishing guardianship and getting assistance with her grandson's disability needs. She was now willing to become a kinship foster care provider. She was told it was too late, that there were time limits on initiating such proceedings. "Don't they understand how hard it is to take a child away from your own daughter, to take away her hope . . . "

An additional frustration reported by the agencies was that being a "client" under one agency (for example, foster care) often prevented obtaining needed services from another agency (for example, trying to access specialized therapy or respite from a disabilities services agency). Some grandparents were reported to have turned down needed kinship foster care financial assistance in order to access disability-related services for their grandchild.

Mutual support groups. Support group leaders told us that they were surprised at the ease with which they were able to convene and manage the support group meetings. Locations included agency offices, schools, a local community center with a playground for the children and, for one set of summer-time group meetings, the outdoor patio of a local laundromat. They agreed that providing respite and transportation enabled grandparents to attend who would not have done so otherwise. Also, scheduling meetings to suit the grandparents' schedules, telephone calls reminding grandparents of the meetings and the transportation arrangements, and providing snacks, and social time at the meetings all helped to encourage good attendance. The leaders reported few missed sessions.

All of the agencies originally intended to hold evening or weekend meetings. However, most found that day time meetings worked better, because the children were usually in school, and grandparents were more open to doing something for themselves during this time. However, one agency did offer an evening group to accommodate grandparents who also worked. This agency provided on-site respite as the grandparents in this group usually preferred to bring their grandchildren with them.

Leaders also commented on the openness of the discussions in the support group meetings, grandparents' willingness to discuss controversial topics like the use of corporal punishment, and how the "taking care of the carer" segment came to be valued by many grandparents as a time when they would give themselves permission to do something for themselves. As one grandmother stated ten minutes into one support group meeting: "When are we doing the deep breathing exercises, that's my favorite part." The groups were treated by many participants as a safe place to talk about their concerns. It was also somewhere where they received support from their peers, and where they acknowledged feeling less alone in their caregiving having found others with the same experience. In addition, many of the grandparents offered specific advice and suggestions to their peers, several were trained as peer volunteers who then accompanied other grandparents to reapply for benefits, and one reconnected with her own training as a counselor and became the co-leader of a support group.

The needs of groups varied and leaders appreciated having a manual that permitted choosing sessions that reflected the interests of a particular group of grandparents. For example, one group made extensive use of the materials on caring for teens. Others did not use this section because the grandparents in the group were all caring for very young children. Leaders also brought in additional material, for example an educational piece on budgeting, to respond to specific needs raised by grandparents. One suggested activity for "taking care of the carer" was advice on proper nutrition. Grandparents were universally uninterested in being told to change what they eat. However, one agency offered fruit and chopped vegetables as a snack at the meetings and provided enough that grandparents often took some of it home, perhaps better achieving the educational piece's intended change.

Need for long-term planning. The project provided for six support group meetings for each grandparent carer and approximately 12 months of case management services. However, agencies routinely continued support group meetings for those who were interested in attending. Agencies were very concerned about how to continue the project's activities and also to assist grandparents to anticipate and prepare for future needs as well as current concerns. Agencies reported playing critical roles in opening discussions about the guardianship status of grandchildren, planning for who would assume care should the grandparent no longer be able, engaging schools and other agencies in facilitating the transition from school to work for older grandchildren, and considering wills, life insurance and other needs. Here the agencies' role in having children declared eligible for developmental disabilities services proved critical. It both offered the opportunity to continue services for the families, and opened up options for future planning.

Follow-up funding. All of the agencies were involved in constant discussions and negotiations with the city's and state's developmental disabilities agencies to secure permanent funding for their grandparent assistance efforts. The state agency, in particular, was very supportive and provided financial assistance as the agencies deemed the children eligible for disability-related services. These funds also provided some support for the administrative expenses associated with aiding grandparents and running the mutual support groups.

DISCUSSION

To the extent that grandparent caregiving is increasingly a normative experience of older years, particularly in urban, low income neighborhoods, the findings derived from this demonstration project suggest that dialogues must be initiated among the varying funding and regulatory agencies to support these families, identify a lead agency, and arrange for shared programs and resources. Only in this way will "helping agencies" help grandparent carers. Of critical concern is the relationship between child protective, foster care, and disability services agencies. The children in these family situations, particularly those involved in abuse and neglect situations, are most vulnerable. The absence of coordinated service delivery, appearances and realities of stigmatizing caregiving grandparents, and the presenting of multiple agency initiated barriers to accessing needed services all contribute to increasing the negative impact of children's disabilities. Coordination with aging agencies is also called for. Grandparents themselves have many needs and appear unwilling to admit to them for fear that children's agencies will remove the child. Involvement of aging agencies will increase the likelihood that the grandparents own needs will be recognized and addressed in a supportive rather than accusatory environment. Social workers are challenged to play critical roles in advocating for and facilitating the dialogues and policy changes that will underpin the successful realization of this service approach.

The absence of funding for grandparent initiatives is also of critical concern. Grandparent caregiving is occurring in an environment in which the resources have already been divided up among client groups and addressing grandparents' needs is seen as taking resources from others. The needs documented here are extensive, needs that in many agencies' minds will require the allocation or reallocation of considerable resources. As Venkatesh (1997) points out, this is not a situation that encourages agencies, particularly well-established agencies with existing clienteles, to seriously pursue providing services to this group. Grandparents' own reluctance and lack of time and resources to speak up for themselves compounds the problem. Finally, the need to traverse children's services, aging services and disability services makes it more difficult for established providers, many of whom already serve only one of these groups, to provide leadership. Social workers must be active in encouraging their agencies to be open to identifying new needs and creative in finding and supporting solutions to newly identified pressing service needs. They should also be open to building relationships and working cooperatively with agencies they would consider non-traditional providers.

This demonstration showed that, at least for these grandparent carers, support groups coupled with an agency willing to do casework and advocate on behalf of their clientele can provide some reassurance and relief to many older adults faced with skip-generation parenting. Experience showed us that many of the grandparents appreciated the attention they received and perhaps just knowing that there was somewhere to turn was helpful. Obviously, many had complex and difficult lives and attendance at a support group did not solve their problems, but the simple reassurance of knowing that others shared their experiences and challenges was helpful.

Grandparent caregiver circumstances suggest a need for agencies that are not bound by existing models of service and established clienteles, have a history and interest in advocacy, listen to and develop services for consumers, understand their communities, and are willing to traverse service systems and develop innovative needed services even with limited resources. These are the characteristics of Venkatesh's mid-tier agencies (1997) and were certainly the profile of the three agencies in this study. As was noted by Janicki, McCallion, Grant-Griffin, and Kolomer (2000), two of the three agencies better fit the model of mid-tier. While all three agencies were successful, the two genuine mid-tiers experienced fewer problems recruiting subjects and gaining their trust. They were seen "as of the community." Also, despite the small amount of money funding their demonstrations, these two agencies at different times involved all of their staff in activities to support the grandparents, creating an "agency family" atmosphere, while the third designated specific staff. Involving mid-tier agencies appeared critical to the project's success. Even if the designated resource and institutional host problems were resolved, the findings suggest that accessibility, sensitivity and trust will continue to be critical to effectively reaching out and serving grandparents. More efforts are needed to understand the role of mid-tier agencies in poor urban communities and how their involvement might improve delivery in other areas of service need.

The project did not involve third tier or grassroots organizations, only legally established not-for-profit agencies, already known to developmental disabilities services and aging agencies. This provided for accountability for the funds given to the agency, and spoke to their ability to negotiate with funders to continue the program's services after the demonstration period. This may have limited the project's ability to reach some grandparents. For example, our experience showed that Latino grandparents proved more difficult to recruit and were often reluctant to complete forms and participate in support group meetings. The three agencies choose to serve these families regardless of their willingness to complete these procedures. However, it is also possible that some grandparents in need, Latino and non-Latino, choose not to enter the project in any way because of these requirements. Workers should recognize that third tier organizations and individuals are an important resource for reaching the most vulnerable and isolated in society. Future research studies should also look at the success of informal grassroots level providers in locating families in need but not otherwise receiving services, and what range of services these families will accept and the providers can offer without risking their grassroots character.

REFERENCES

Axelson, J.A. (1993). *Counseling and Development in a Multicultural Society* (2nd ed.). Pacific Grove, CA: Brooks/Cole Publishing Co.

Barnhill, S. (1996). Three generations at risk: Imprisoned women, their children, and grandmother caregivers. *Generations, 20*, (1), 39-40.

Burton, L.M. (1992). Black grandparents rearing grandchildren of drug-addicted parents: Stressors, outcomes, and social service needs. *The Gerontologist, 32*, (6), 744-751.

Crumbley, J., & Little, R. (Eds.) (1997). *Relatives Raising Children: An Overview of Kinship Care*. Washington, DC: Child Welfare League of America.

Fuller-Thomson, E., Minkler, M., & Driver, D. (1997). A profile of grandparents raising grandchildren in the US. *The Gerontologist, 37*, (3), 406-411.

Grandparent Resource Center. (1998a). *The Grandparent Raising Grandchildren Book: Support Services Resource Guide.* New York, NY: New York City Department for the Aging.

Grandparent Resource Center. (1998b). *For Grandparents Raising Grandchildren: A Series of Workshops to Help you COPE.* New York, NY: New York City Department for the Aging.

Gratton, B., & Wilson, V. (1988). Family support systems and the minority elderly: A cautionary analysis. *Journal of Gerontological Social Work, 13*, (1-2), 81-93.

Harden, A.W., Clark, R., and Maguire, K. (1997). *Informal and formal kinship care.* Report for the Office of the Assistant Secretary for Planning and Evaluation (Task Order HHS-100-95-0021). Washington, DC: U.S. Department of Health and Human Services.

Henderson, J.N., Gutierrez-Mayka, M., Garcia, J., and Boyd, S. (1993). Model for Alzheimer's disease support group development in African-American and Hispanic populations. *Gerontologist, 33*, (3), 409-414.

Iglehart, A.P., and Becerra, R.M. (1996). Social work and the ethnic agency: A history of neglect. *Journal of Multicultural Social Work, 4*, (1), 1-20.

Jendrek, M.P. (1994). Grandparents who parent their grandchildren: Circumstances and decisions. *The Gerontologist, 34*, (2), 206-216.

Kolomer, S. (2000). Kinship foster care and its impact on grandmother caregivers. *Journal of Gerontological Studies.*

Lockery, S.A. (1991). Family and social supports: Caregiving among racial and ethnic minority elders. *Generations, 15*, (4), 58-62.

McCallion, P., Janicki, M.P., and Grant-Griffin, L. (1997). Exploring the impact of culture and acculturation on older families caregiving for persons with developmental disabilities. *Family Relations, 46*, (4), 347-357.

McCallion, P., and Tobin, S. (1995). Social worker orientations to permanency planning by older parents caring at home for sons and daughters with developmental disabilities. *Mental Retardation, 33*(3), 153-162.

Minkler, M., Driver, D., Roe, K.M., and Bedeian, K. (1993). Community interventions to support grandparent caregivers. *The Gerontologist, 33*, (6), 807-811.

Minkler, M., Roe, K.M., and Price, M. (1992). The physical and emotional health of grandmothers raising grandchildren in the crack cocaine epidemic. *The Gerontologist, 32*, (6), 752-761.

Sakauye, K. (1989). Ethnic variations in family support of the frail elderly. In M.Z. Goldstein, (Ed.). *Family Involvement in Treatment of the Frail Elderly.* (pp. 63-106). Washington, DC: American Psychiatric Press.

Samuel Sadin Institute on Law. (1997a). *Help for Grandparent Caregivers: A Guide to Legal Custody, Foster Care, Kinship Foster Care, Guardianship, Standby Guardianship, Adoption (Vol. I).* New York, NY: Brookdale Center on Aging of Hunter College.

Samuel Sadin Institute on Law. (1997b). *Help for Grandparent Caregivers: A Guide to Visitation, Housing, Education, Medical Consent (Vol. II).* New York, NY: Brookdale Center on Aging of Hunter College.

Samuel Sadin Institute on Law. (1998). *Help for Grandparent Caregivers: A Guide to the Family Assistance Program, New York State's Temporary Assistance to Needy Families Program (TANF) (Vol. III)*. New York, NY: Brookdale Center on Aging Hunter College.

Strawbridge, W.J., Wallhagen, M.I., Shema, S.J., and Kaplan, G.A. (1997). New burdens or more of the same? Comparing grandparent, spouse, and adult child caregivers. *Gerontologist, 37*, (4), 505-510.

Sung, K.T. (1995). Measures and dimensions of filial piety in Korea. *Gerontologist, 35*, (2), 240-247.

Venkatesh, S.A. (1997). The three-tier model: How helping occurs in urban, poor communities. *Social Service Review*, 574-606.

Zambrana, R.E. (1991). Cross-cultural methodological strategies in the study of low income racial ethnic populations. In H. Hibbard, P.A. Nutting, and M.L. Grady (Eds.), *Primary Care Research: Theory and Methods* (pp. 221-227) USDHHS, Public Health Service, Agency for Health Care Policy and Research Pub. No. 91-0011, Rockville, MD.

Kinship Foster Care
and Its Impact
on Grandmother Caregivers

Stacey R. Kolomer, CSW

SUMMARY. Kinship foster care programs are designed to address the needs of relatives, usually grandparents, who have taken in children who have been removed from their homes voluntarily, or following a substantiated report of neglect and/or abuse. The author reviews the history of kinship foster care nationally and examines related research. Reported are findings on a survey of kinship foster care programs nationwide and from qualitative interviews with nine grandmothers from New York City who were kinship foster care providers. Particular attention was paid in these surveys to the impact of kinship foster care on families caring for children with disabilities. *[Article copies available for a fee from The Haworth Document Delivery Service: 1-800-342-9678. E-mail address: <getinfo@haworthpressinc.com> Website: <http://www.HaworthPress.com>]*

KEYWORDS. History of kinship foster care, kinship care research, survey of programs, impact on caregiving families, special needs children, regrets of grandparents

---

Stacey R. Kolomer is a Doctoral Candidate, School of Social Welfare, University at Albany.

Address correspondence to: Stacey R. Kolomer, CSW, School of Social Welfare, University at Albany, 135 Western Avenue, Albany, NY 12222 (E-mail: merini@aol.com).

Funding for this project was provided by the Joseph P. Kennedy, Jr. Foundation and by an NASW Jane Aron Doctoral Fellowship.

[Haworth co-indexing entry note]: "Kinship Foster Care and Its Impact on Grandmother Caregivers." Kolomer, Stacey R. Co-published simultaneously in *Journal of Gerontological Social Work* (The Haworth Press, Inc.) Vol. 33, No. 3, 2000, pp. 85-102; and: *Grandparents as Carers of Children with Disabilities: Facing the Challenges* (ed: Philip McCallion and Matthew Janicki) The Haworth Press, Inc., 2000, pp. 85-102. Single or multiple copies of this article are available for a fee from The Haworth Document Delivery Service [1-800-342-9678, 9:00 a.m. - 5:00 p.m. (EST). E-mail address: getinfo@haworthpressinc.com].

Kinship foster care programs at both the federal and state levels are designed to address the needs of relatives, usually grandparents, who have taken in children who have been removed from their homes following a substantiated report of neglect and/or abuse. In some cases it is extended to children for whom parents have relinquished responsibility in other circumstances. Among these children are individuals with developmental disabilities and other special needs (Dubowitz, Feigelman, Harrington, Starr, & Zuravin, 1994). An unanticipated rise in the number of children needing out-of-home placement has expanded the use of kinship foster care, leading to a dramatic increase in grandparents having to take on the role as caregivers to their grandchildren. Across the country states have been struggling to design appropriate programs for kin who have taken on the role as primary caregiver to children. Less attention has been paid to the unique needs of grandparents caring for grandchildren with developmental disabilities.

Since a large majority of kinship foster care providers are grandmothers, this paper focuses on how this population is affected by kinship foster care programs. The literature review outlines (1) the history of kinship foster care; (2) goals of both federal and state kinship foster care programs; (3) rights, responsibilities, and consequences for kin providers, and (4) existing research about kinship foster care and its impact on grandparents. Findings are reported on a survey of state kinship foster care programs and from interviews with grandmothers who are currently or have been in the past kinship foster care parents. Special attention in these surveys was paid to the impact of kinship foster care on families caring for children with disabilities (Dubowitz et al., 1994). Finally, recommendations are offered for the future of kinship foster care and how it might better impact on the needs of grandchildren with developmental disabilities and other special needs.

KINSHIP FOSTER CARE

History of Kinship Foster Care

In many states kinship foster care follows the traditional foster care model replacing non-relatives with relatives of the children as caregivers. Nationwide there are approximately 500,000 children currently residing in a formal kinship foster care setting (Scannapieco et al., 1997). For many years states have placed children who have been neglected and/or abused with relatives. Originally there was a reluctance on the part of child welfare agencies to place children with relatives for fear of generational abuse and the belief that families are trapped in a cycle of violence (Jackson, 1999). In 1979, the Supreme Court determined that relatives could not be excluded from the definition of foster parents qualifying for federal benefits (Berrick, Barth, and Needell, 1994; Crumbley & Little, 1997). The Adoption Assistance and Child Welfare Act of 1980 (P.L. 96-272) required that a child who is in need of an out-of-home placement be placed in the least restrictive setting (Dubo-witiz et al., 1994; Gleeson, 1999). States interpreted the federal guideline for the least restrictive setting as "family-like"and thus encouraged placement of children with kin. The Adoption and Safe Families Act of 1997 amended the earlier act by adding financial incentives for adoption and defined "least restrictive setting" as accessing children's kin as the primary option for placement (Genty, 1998). The end result was that states increasingly relied on kin to provide homes to children removed from their parents' or guardians' care.

Between 1985 and 1990 there was a 27 percent decrease in available traditional foster homes while the number of children needing out-of-home placement increased by 47 percent (Scannapieco et al., 1996; Davidson, 1997). There were a number of reasons for both of these trends. First, the availability of traditional foster families declined due to scandals and con-cerns associated with the foster care system, an increase in the number of women entering the workforce, and low reimbursement for providing care (Ingram, 1996). Yet, as the availability of foster families declined, the num-ber of reports of child abuse and/or neglect increased (Dubowitz et al., 1994). Additionally, stigmatizing social problems which jeopardize the integrity of families such as AIDS, teen pregnancy, homelessness, substance abuse, and poverty also dramatically increased, leading to more children needing out-of-home placements (Scannapieco et al., 1996; Davidson, 1997). Between 1985 and 1990 there was only a 20 percent increase in the number of children placed in traditional foster care placements, in contrast to the 200 percent increase of children placed with kin (Zwas, 1992). Urban areas have had particularly dramatic rises in the use of kin as foster care families. In Balti-more, Maryland 75 percent of all children needing out of home care were placed with kin (Curtis, Boyd, Leipold, & Petit, 1995). In New York City half of the foster care population is placed with relatives (Green Book, 1998).

Goals of Kinship Foster Care

The overt goal of using kin as foster care providers was to address the "least restrictive setting" requirement of the Adoption Assistance and Child Welfare Act of 1980 (Dubowitz et al., 1994; Gleeson, 1999). Using kin gives children the possibility to continue to live in a familiar setting (Davidson, 1997). A bond with kin already exists for the child and no new relationship needs to be established during a turbulent time in the child's life (Hornby, Zeller, & Karraker, 1996). Placing a child with a relative allows the parent to have frequent contact with the child, which can facilitate long term goals of reunification and family preservation (Dubowitz et al., 1994; Hornby et al., 1996). Relatives are more likely to be invested in the growth and development of a child placed in their care than non-relatives would (Scannapieco et al., 1996). A child in kinship foster care is also less likely to be uprooted and transferred to another home, which frequently occurs with children in traditional foster care placements (Scannapieco et al., 1997). In the past it was often difficult to find foster families willing to adopt children with disabilities. Greater reliance on kin has eased difficulties in finding placements and reduced the likelihood of placements failing. Finally, children in kinship foster care are usually in an environment that supports their cultural and ethnic identity (Scannapieco et al., 1996).

Rights, Responsibilities, and Consequences

Kinship foster care has been administered as a selective program. The benefits are means tested as the children's family of origin in the past had to be eligible for Aid to Families with Dependent Children now Temporary Assistance for Needy Families for the kinship foster families to receive the monthly stipend for the child (Child Welfare League of America, 1994). Benefits are provided to the kin caregivers on a monthly basis. The stipend is intended to provide a child with adequate food, shelter, clothing, and other necessities. Children who are in kinship foster homes receive medical coverage under Medicaid. The families are also eligible to receive in-kind services such as respite care and case management.

The family receives a monthly stipend for every child in care. The amount of the stipend varies depending on the state, the child's age, and if the child is classified as medically fragile. As the child ages, the stipend increases. Counties within states may offer different stipends to their residents. For example, in New York upstate counties a caregiver of a two-year-old child received $367 per month, while a New York City resident received $401 for a two-year-old child in 1996 (Green Book, 1998). Many states also provide higher stipend rates to children who are diagnosed as medically fragile. In Baltimore, Maryland a family caring for a child without specialized medical needs receives $550, while a family caring for a medically fragile child receives almost triple the usual stipend rate (Payne-Wells, 1999). All kinship foster care children are covered by Medicaid for health insurance. Although eligible for all of these benefits, in practice, due to the length of the evaluation process children are often in care for several months before any assistance is received. The decision to provide back payments to families in such situations is up to the local administrator.

This approach to kinship foster care payments does permit a level of consumer sovereignty, since the families receive cash and can choose how they wish to spend it. However, the program also exercises social control. A case worker monitors the family to insure that the children's basic needs are being met. If it is determined that children are not receiving adequate food, shelter, or clothing, the child can be removed from the care of kin or the stipend can be reduced until the needs are being met to the satisfaction of the foster care agency.

Nationally it is not known how many children in kinship foster care have disabilities. The label "special needs" is given to a range of categories including children belonging to large sibling groups and minorities (Curtis et al., 1995). This leaves children who have developmental disabilities, but who are not classified as medically fragile, and their carers at risk because their specific needs are not being recognized and addressed. Yet, children in kinship foster care are at high risk for disabilities since prior to placement these children were often exposed to risk factors that left them vulnerable. These risk factors include, but are not limited to, abuse, neglect, prenatal exposure to alcohol and drugs, poverty, and lack of prenatal care. Dysfunctional families are also less likely to have taken steps to ensure that disabilities are identified.

There are also factors which place additional stress on kinship caregivers and encourage them to not pursue benefits to which they may be entitled. This adds to the burdens of caring for a child with a disability. One concern is that kinship foster care providers often experience criticism by others. If a child is removed from the home due to neglect and/or abuse and is then placed with a kin provider, such as a grandmother, the entire family must cope with society's judgements. Although the idea that family violence occurs in cycles and repeats across generations has been discounted, many people still blame the whole family when abuse occurs (Jackson, 1999). The same sense of blame is often attached to extended families when the reason for placement is substance abuse, AIDS/HIV, or imprisonment. Grandmothers who are caring for children who have developmental disabilities may feel especially vulnerable to criticism, as often the developmental disabilities are attributable to the risk factors the children were exposed to in the care of their parents.

Secondly, kinship caregivers report a lack of understanding about why they need assistance to provide for their own relatives. Kinship care providers are often questioned by others about their motives for taking in kin. They are criticized for taking government funds for caring for their own family members as the care provided is often viewed by others as their moral responsibility (Crumbley & Little, 1997). People also question why kinship care providers should receive additional services such as respite and case management. Doubt about the sincerity of their caregiving and a sense of being judged by others causes additional stress for an already overwhelmed family (Mandelbaum, 1995). In such circumstances, grandmothers raising children who have developmental disabilities may feel additionally isolated by the overwhelming needs of the child and the lack of understanding by others. All of this suggests that kinship foster care providers are at least under different, if not additional, pressures than traditional providers, and that those caring for children with developmental disabilities may be especially under strain, yet state by state there is great variation in the recognition of these unique needs.

Finally, guilt, embarrassment, anger, and resentment are all common reactions of kin care providers (Crumbley & Little, 1997). Since grandmothers are most often the providers of care, questions about their own parenting of the grandchild's parent are asked. Grandmothers may also resent being a caregiver again when they have reached a time in their lives when they are ready to settle down (Crumbley & Little, 1997). They may also be angry at the foster care agency for intruding on their lives. For example, caregivers who have previously raised children may feel insulted at the idea of being required to attend parenting classes (Crumbley & Little, 1997). Overall becoming a kinship foster care provider causes many mixed feelings and emotions within the grandparent.

Programs for Kin Caregivers Across the Country

Foster care programs are subsidized by the federal government if they are in compliance with Title IV-E of the Social Security Act, but decisions about where to place children are up to the individual states. To gain insight into what programs are available for kinship care providers telephone contact and electronic mail were exchanged with a random sample of twelve states' child welfare agencies. Inquiries were made about the number of kinship foster families in each state, the services and funding available to the families, the requirements to become a kinship foster provider, and services available to the families in kinship foster care who are caring for a child who has a developmental disability.

Overall, the findings suggest that there is a broad continuum of service approaches whose variation appears to be rarely driven by the children's or kin caregivers' needs. In several states kin receive the same services and are mandated to fulfill the same requirements as non relative foster care homes. Other states have chosen not to allow kin to receive foster care funds, and families without other resources must apply for funding from Temporary Assistance for Needy Families. The families, therefore, receive significantly lower financial support than traditional foster families. Still other states have in place or are presently creating innovative programs to support kin caring for children who are in the custody of the State. These ambitious states have recognized that care by family members is different from that provided by non-relative caregivers. The programs they have developed recognize that kin caregivers have distinct needs that need to be addressed through more creative program options.

For example, one option that 23 of the 24 counties in Maryland have chosen is a program for kin that allows families more independence and less formal supervision, although the children remain wards of the state. The families who participate receive a stipend that is less than what foster care home providers would receive, but is more than TANF. The home inspection is done informally. The family is visited once every two months by a caseworker rather than once a month. The caregivers are not required to participate in mandatory parenting and caregiving classes as is required for traditional foster parents. A family that has a child who has a disability receives a stipend at a higher rate.

Four states interviewed are part of a ten state group (Alaska, Colorado, Massachusetts, South Dakota, Hawaii, Illinois, Nebraska, New Mexico, California, and Washington) that have used their own funds to establish subsidized kin guardianship programs (Takas & Hegar, 1999). Subsidized guardianship enables kin, rather than the state, to have authority over the children being cared for, and still receive a stipend for providing care (Zwas, 1992). Parental rights are maintained unless it is determined that it is not in the best interest of the child. Reports from respondents suggest that kinship guardianship programs are more cost effective than other options (Zwas, 1992). They also indicated that relative caregivers report no longer feeling pressured to adopt the child. Several other responding states indicated they have applied for federal waivers to undertake similar subsidized guardianship demonstration projects (Takas et al., 1999).

Some states also reported looking at other innovative ways to address permanency planning. Although the use of kin caregivers has helped states with achieving least restrictive setting, since the introduction of the Safe Families Adoption Act, states have been struggling to find permanent homes for children who have been in foster care for more than six months. Respondents stated kin are often reluctant to adopt their own family members because of the ties to the child's parent. As a result agencies feel forced to warn families that they may lose rights to care for the child if they do not adopt. One state, Kentucky, is currently developing a project in three counties in which family members would not commit to adoption but instead to permanent custody. With permanent custody the family can continue to receive a subsidy. It was also reported that this program involved less costly court processes as kin are able to represent themselves.

Additionally, interviews with state foster care agencies indicated that families caring for children with developmental disabilities usually do receive higher monthly stipends. However, there does not appear to be any consistency as to how such children with special needs receive services from state to state or even within states. In some states, for example Florida, children who have disabilities receive services from specialized foster care agencies contracted by the state (personal communication, Tonie White, June 22, 1999). Other States permit families to obtain services from the developmental disabilities service providers, but often there are long wait lists for such services. Finally, some states believe that it is up to the assigned public or private foster care agency to insure that children receive any specialized services needed. However, some respondents acknowledged that this approach means that some children with developmental disabilities do not receive adequate, specialized, early intervention services, and grandparents are often forced to pay for such services themselves, if they are even able to access them.

The interviews with staff of state child welfare agencies suggests that across the country, there are states that are developing innovative programs to help grandparents with their role as caregiver to their grandchildren. Less is reported to be happening on a national level. With the exception of discussion of grandparent caregivers at several White House Conferences on Aging and some legislative initiatives that have not passed, respondents suggest that the federal government has been slow to respond to the specific needs of grandparent caregivers. It was also acknowledged that most states have been reluctant to address the specific needs of grandparents caring for grandchildren with developmental disabilities. Interviews conducted with grandparent caregivers appear to support the view that these carers lack critical support from local, state, and national agencies.

Interviews with Kinship Foster Care Providers

An opportunity to interview grandparents in kinship foster care who are caring for a child with a developmental disability occurred in a larger study of caregiving grandparents (McCallion, Janicki, Grant-Griffin, & Kolomer, 2000). Grandparents who were part of the formal kinship foster care system presented themselves as being in a dissimilar situation than their peers who were informally caring for their grandchildren. Many reported that although they were satisfied with the additional income provided to them by the foster care system, they felt very limited in the services they could access that would benefit the children they were caring for. These statements motivated additional questions about kinship foster care and what were the available services for children with developmental disabilities.

Sample: Telephone interviews were conducted with nine grandparent caregivers living in New York City. All of the participants currently or in the past have been kinship foster caregivers. Seven were grandmothers to the children they cared for and two were grandaunts. Eight were African American and one identified herself as Caucasian. None of the participants were currently married. Seven of the participants were over 60 years old and two were younger than 60. This profile is consistent with many other reports of grandparent carers (see for example, Burnette, 1999; McCallion, Janicki, Grant-Griffin, & Kolomer, 2000). All but one of the families were caring for more than one child, with one grandaunt caring for six of her nieces and nephews. In addition, all of the grandparents interviewed were caring for at least one grandchild who was diagnosed with a developmental disability.

The initial contact was made by the community agency working with the grandmother or grandaunt. The kinship foster care provider then gave permission to the community agency to release her phone number to the researcher.

Method: A semi-structured telephone interview was completed with each grandparent. The interview lasted approximately 45 minutes. The protocol (see Table 1) consisted of 16 primary questions such as: How did you become a kinship foster care parent and Does your child with a disability receive additional services from kinship foster care? These were supplemented with 22 follow up questions, for example, a response of "yes" to "Does your child with a disability receive additional services from kinship foster care," resulted in the following supplementary question: What are those services and how often does the child receive those services? The questions can be found in Table 1. Extensive notes were taken during the interview. The majority of the questions were open-ended, and a semi-structured approach to the interviews was chosen to elicit richer detail from the participants. This also permitted the researcher to make comparisons of their experiences using a cross comparative grounded theory approach to identify common themes (Fortune & Reid, 1999; Tutty, Rothery, & Grinnell, 1996).

Grandparents acknowledged the importance of the assistance they receive from the foster care system. As one grandmother put it, "I don't know if I could manage without the money or having someone to talk to." However, the general impression reported by the grandmothers of being in the foster care system was that it is a negative experience. Most of the grandmothers reported that foster care agencies failed to provide needed services for the children such as psychological assessments and counseling. Especially lacking were interventions and services for children identified as having developmental disabilities. Several grandmothers discussed the lengthy waits and long distances they traveled for appointments and evaluations. Indeed, some grandmothers indicated that they preferred not to be connected to the foster care system, but acknowledged they remained because they needed the stipend for the survival of the family. Common concerns and experiences were identified in the following areas: Becoming a foster care parent, home evaluations, services and funding received from the foster care agency, parent training courses, experiences with the foster care agency after the children

TABLE 1. Interview Questions for Kinship Foster Grandparent Caregivers

1. How did you become a foster care parent?
2. Who came to your home? 2a. Did you know they were coming?
3. What types of questions did they ask you? 3a. Were you offered a choice of whether you wanted to care for your grandchild(ren) without being a kinship foster care parent?
4. Did a caseworker look over your home when the children were brought to you? 4a. How was the evaluation process explained to you? 4b. What types of things did he/she say he/she was looking for?
5. Did you need any additional furniture when your grandchildren came to live with you? 5a. If yes, were you offered assistance in getting the furniture? 5b. Have you received any additional furniture from the foster care agency?
6. Were you offered any services during this initial visit? 6a. What were those services? 6b. How frequently are you receiving those services?
7. After the children were placed in your home how soon were you contacted by the foster care agency after the initial visit?
8. Was your home reevaluated? 8a. How was the evaluation process explained to you?
9. After the second evaluation were you told that anything else was needed in your home? 9a. How were you assisted by the foster care agency to get what you needed for your home?
10. What types of services were you offered? 10a. Did you need these services? 10b. If yes, are you receiving these services? 10c. How often? 10d. Are they helpful?
11. Do you receive respite services? 11a. If yes, how frequently?
12. Does your child with a disability receive additional services from kinship foster care? 12a. If yes, what were these services? 12b. How often does the child receive these services?
13. Were you offered any parent training courses? 13a. If yes, have you attended these classes? 13b. How helpful are these classes? 13c. What was the focus in these classes?
14. How soon after you became a kinship foster care parent did you receive the stipend?
15. Does this income cover all of the child's expenses? 15a. If no, how do you cover the expenses of your grandchild?
16. How available is your case manager? 16a. How often do you have contact with your case manager?

were placed in the home, and special services needed for children with developmental disabilities.

Becoming a kinship foster parent. Mrs. Z reported hearing from a neighbor that her daughter had given birth. Knowing that her daughter's substance abuse and mental illness made her unable to provide a stable environment for the child, Mrs. Z and her husband requested to take the child home upon discharge from the hospital. Mrs. Z was told by the hospital social worker to go to family court. After nine months and $2,000 in legal fees Mrs. Z was able to bring her grandchild home to live with her.

Many of the grandmothers interviewed became kinship caregivers when they were contacted by the hospital requesting that they bring home their newborn grandchild because the infant was born drug addicted. One grandmother reported never being informed of the child's health status or why she was being asked to take the child. Most of the participants were surprised to become caregivers to their grandchildren. Each reported they had to become certified as kinship foster care parents. One grandmother had requested to care for the children when they were initially removed but was refused until her home became certified. The children were placed in a traditional foster care home outside of their neighborhood. It took one month for her to get the children in her home. Another grandmother was asked by the city's Department of Social Services to take the grandchild but was never informed that she could be a kinship foster care parent and receive a higher stipend than TANF. She then had to appeal to the courts to allow her to become a kinship foster parent.

The caregivers were quite open to discussing why the parents were unable to be responsible for their own children. Several of the parents were active substance abusers. Two had dual diagnoses of mental illness and substance abuse.

Home Evaluation. Mrs. L was told she needed separate beds to care for her five grandchildren. Since the foster care agency she was working with did not offer assistance, Mrs. L had to take the children with her to look for extra beds and furniture at the Salvation Army or in the street. "I would scrub those beds until they looked new."

Most grandmothers reported that they were given no warning when the caseworker came to evaluate the home. Frequently on the first visit the caseworker would open the cabinets to ensure that there was food in the home, investigate if window guards were installed, inspect fire alarms, and check the condition of the furniture, especially beds. If any of these items were missing or broken, the grandparent was told to fix it before the next evaluation which would follow in one month. Seven grandparents reported that they were expected to acquire any missing items on their own; no assistance was offered to obtain any of these items. Obtaining the needed items was difficult for the grandmothers as their funds were limited. Two grandmothers were provided with extra beds for the children.

One grandmother reported that she was told she needed to move from her one bedroom apartment because it was too small for her and the four children she was caring for. When the caseworker returned in one month and the family had not yet moved, the grandmother was found not to qualify as a kinship foster parent. She was unable to get benefits from kinship foster care, but the children remained in the home. She eventually had to go to court to be reevaluated and receive back payments.

Services and Funding: Ms. G took in her sister's grandson who was diagnosed as having autism. Her sister cared for his four siblings. Mrs. G made the decision to leave the foster care system because she was unable to get her grand nephew into the specialized programs he needed. She reported that the money may have covered his basic needs but it was not enough for him to have a tutor, join an after-school program, or go to summer camp.

Many of grandmothers reported a lag time from the time they received the children in their homes until the first foster care payment check was received. Most stated they received the first check between one to two months following the placement of the child. One grandmother reported not receiving a check for two years because the agency did not feel she had sufficient space to care for the children, although they left the children in her care. Although stipends were usually awarded with retroactive payments, many of the caregivers reported that they had difficulty managing before the payment came. One grandmother expressed that it was a hardship that the children did not have desperately needed appropriate clothing.

All of the grandmothers acknowledged that the stipend normally covered all of the children's needs when it was received. Some exceptions were when the children needed additional clothing for the summer or for school. Then the caregivers had to provide additional money through their own finances. One grandmother reported that she purposefully only purchased uniforms for school to cut costs.

One grandmother in this group did receive respite services and another had a home attendant for four hours a day for five days a week. None of the other grandmothers reported being offered services at the time they began to care for the children, but felt such services were justified by the special needs of some of their grandchildren.

Parent Training: "I missed my classes and my funding was reduced. I have begun to attend classes again but no one seems to know when my funding will be reestablished."

All of the caregivers except one had participated in workshops as mandated by the foster care agency. The classes attended focused primarily on behavior management and child care. The caregivers also attended classes that concentrated on their children's specific diagnosis. The classes were described as helpful and interesting. Most of the caregivers reported learning a lot from these workshops. One caregiver reported trying to attend as many classes as possible to further help herself.

The caregivers reported that they were told if they did not attend classes the stipend they receive for the children would be cut. Many of the carers reported difficulties in maintaining attendance at classes due to lack of transportation to the classes, the inconvenience of the schedule, and finding particular classes already closed when they tried to register. The providers also commented that due to regulations of the foster care agency several topics, such as behavior management, had to be repeated despite attending the class in the past.

After the children were placed in your home: Mrs. J complained "My foster care agency moved last month and I do not know how to get in contact with them."

All of the care providers reported that they are visited once a month by their caseworker and four stated that they stay in regular contact with their worker. One common thread in the interviews was that each of the caregivers have had several caseworkers during their time as care providers. Several complained that once they became comfortable with one worker, he or she would leave the position. The carers found it difficult and intrusive to be expected to tell and retell their family history to each new worker. Additionally, with each case worker came a new fear of how actions and behaviors may be interpreted. They expressed concerns that new case workers would negatively view the care they were providing to the children in their care. Grandparents reported feeling stressed by the constant scrutiny of strangers.

Special services for children with developmental disabilities. Three of Mrs. D's grandchildren were diagnosed as having developmental and emotional disabilities. Her foster care agency promised to send the children for psychiatric services but to date no services have been provided.

Most of the caregivers reported not receiving any additional services for children with disabilities. Some were expected to seek services on their own with the additional foster care payments they receive for caring for a child who has a developmental disability. One grandmother stated that her child was sent for counseling at a contracted agency that was out of her area so it was difficult for her to follow-up on his treatment. Another family was sent to specialized hospitals to receive services for the child. Transportation was provided to access these services. All were frustrated by not being able to access local disability related services although there were agencies providing such services in their neighborhoods. However, such agencies were part of the disability, not the foster care network, and could not be accessed by kinship foster care providers.

DISCUSSION AND RECOMMENDATIONS

Much of what was reported by the caregivers is consistent with what has been reported in the literature. These grandmothers felt overwhelmed and discouraged by the lack of support received from the foster care agencies. They also felt judged by the foster care agencies, similar to complaints voiced by other grandparents about society in general (Crumbley & Little, 1997). Additional studies are needed that focus more specifically on the needs of kinship foster families caring for children with developmental disabilities to confirm if the experiences reported by these grandparents are common to others in similar situations. Such research should be conducted with kinship foster care families throughout the country, as each state's unique programs impact on the kinship foster care population differently.

Properly developed, kinship foster care offers children with developmental disabilities who are no longer able to live with their parents (an otherwise hard to place population), the option to live in a familiar, culturally appropriate stable family situation. However, even such supportive families cannot adequately meet these children's needs if special needs are not assessed, and needed supportive services are not easily accessed. Grandparents often face overwhelming financial burdens and application of regulations designed for non-relative caregivers violate the sense of family that the related policies claim they are designed to enhance. Furthermore, these family situations offer the best hope of true permanency for many of these children, but contemplating the termination of parental rights is painful for many grandparents, and adoption means fewer supports, particularly for low income grandparents caring for grandchildren with substantial developmental disabilities. The development of appropriate, consistent policies and services is called for, but the findings reported here suggest that more information is needed before appropriate policies can be developed.

Recommendations for Foster Care Agencies

Programs for grandparents who are kinship care providers need to be delivered on a more consistent basis. Many states have excellent services available to these families, but carers are not aware of them. One recommendation is that foster care agencies have a systematic method of informing carers of what services are available. Formal assessment of the problems experienced by these families is also needed (Gilbert & Terrell, 1998). For example, there are no published reports of how many kinship foster families are caring for children who have special health needs. A more comprehensive assessment of these families by each state is needed to develop appropriate interventions. Having a fuller understanding of how grandparents and grandchildren are affected by being part of the child welfare system will also lead to more appropriate policy development.

States participating in kin guardianship and kin adoption demonstration projects are advancing our knowledge of how to pursue permanency for these families, but the outcomes of these programs are not yet known. Answers to the following questions are needed if states are to be influenced to try similar programs and a comprehensive approach developed. Are the demonstration projects working? How are the families who have participated in these programs functioning? What are the long term effects on the children and the carers? There is also a need for demonstrations that target children with disabilities. Information must first be gathered on numbers of children involved and how children who have developmental disabilities are faring in kinship foster care system. Information is also needed on what types of services are available to these children.

To make changes within the kinship foster care program it is important to also consider how the system functions. One strong message from the grandparents was that they are frustrated with the constant new assignment of caseworkers. It is well documented that child welfare workers have high caseloads and many burnout (Drake & Yamada, 1996). After developing ties to caseworkers, grandparents very often find themselves starting over after short periods of time. Retelling the stories of their lives and helping workers understand their family situation can be stressful for this group of caregivers. Kinship foster families would benefit from having more consistency in their relationships with their foster care agencies. For families who have children with developmental disabilities it is particularly important that the child's condition be clearly understood. Consistency is essential to the growth and development for any child, but especially one who already has many obstacles to overcome. Exploration of how the position of child welfare worker can be more valued, and consideration of how to make the job more attractive so that people may stay longer demands attention.

Kinship families caring for children with developmental disabilities need special examination. As expressed by the grandparents and confirmed by the information provided by various states, services for these families is inconsistent and sporadic. For all children, but especially those with developmental disabilities, early intervention is necessary for children to thrive. These children also need dependable medical attention, schooling, and interventions. These services exist in the disabilities service system in most states. However, some states in their interpretation of state and federal legislation appear to have determined that children with developmental disabilities already receiving services in the foster care system may not access services from disability providers. Foster care agencies already face many resource challenges. It may be too much, and not a good use of resources to ask them to duplicate services.

Not yet addressed in these recommendations are grandparents who are informally providing care for grandchildren. More information is needed on the numbers of grandparents who are informally caring for their grandchildren and the scope of the responsibilities and concerns that confront them. Interviews with grandparents conducted for this study found instances where grandparents interested in and otherwise eligible for kinship foster care support were denied access by apparently arbitrary regulatory procedures. Also, some of the grandparents avoided or withdrew from kinship foster care because of the misunderstandings about the programs, fear for the integrity of their family, or barriers posed participation in the program for accessing other needed services. Consideration of possible changes in kinship foster care needs to incorporate these perspectives.

Implications for Social Workers

It is frequently stressed by policy makers that children are highly valued in this society. Yet when it comes to their care it appears that "adequacy" is the value applied for children who have been removed from their homes. As agents of change it is up to social workers to advocate for these children and their grandparent caregivers. As the providers of direct services to this growing population it is also up to social workers to make the public aware of the issues these caregivers are dealing with, and of the need for policy changes.

Kinship foster care was created to respond to the lack of traditional foster homes and the increase in children needing out-of-home care. However, social workers must increase understanding that expansion in the use of kinship foster families is not a "second best" option. Such families meet children's needs for established bonds and limit the trauma when a child is removed from the home. Such removals are particularly traumatic for children with disabilities who may not be able to understand what is happening around them. A child's own extended family provides an ideal environment for maintaining a child's identity and preserves cultural and ethnic identity.

The promotion of kinship foster care must become a valued activity in the practice of social work. As part of this promotion social workers should become involved with kinship families on both a micro and macro level. In addition to the assessment of concrete needs, families need to have their emotional needs examined. The introduction of new members into a home will cause strong feelings and changes within the family system. These changes need to be addressed for the family to successfully function as a unit.

At a macro level social workers need to be involved with decisions about policies for these families, as well as creating new programs which would more effectively meet the needs of grandparent caregivers of children with developmental disabilities. Follow up studies are necessary to understand the impact of the innovative programs that are occurring nationwide for grandparent caregivers. Following the publication of successful efforts, states that have been slower to respond to the needs of kinship foster families need to consider duplicating these programs. Social workers can be leaders in advocating for these changes at local, state, and national levels.

Social workers also have responsibility to advocate for the services and information kinship foster caregivers such as grandparents need to care effectively for grandchildren with developmental and other disabilities. It is unreasonable to "forget" that these family caregivers have the same issues and needs as caregivers who are not related to a child. Social workers' unique professional values can assist in the development of policies that address the needs of grandparent caregivers who are providing formal care to their grandchildren. Formal assessments of families' needs, advocating for appropriate services, and providing on going support are all roles which can be fulfilled by social workers.

Without the development of policies that specifically address the needs of grandparent caregivers, social workers will continue to work with a population that is at high risk for financial difficulties, and physical and mental health problems. Social workers working in the foster care system, have important opportunities to make critical differences in the lives of grandparent caregivers and the children for whom they care.

BIBLIOGRAPHY

Bell, W. & Garner, J. (1996). Kincare. *Journal of Gerontological Social Work, 25*(1/2), 489-501.

Berrick, J. D., Barth, Richard P., & Needles, B. (1994). A Comparison of Kinship Foster Homes and Family Foster Homes: Implications for Kinship Foster Care as Family Preservation. *Children and Youth Services Review, 16*(1/2), 33-63.

Child Welfare League of America. (1994). *Kinship Care: A Natural Bridge.* Washington, DC: Child Welfare League of America.

Crumbley, J., & Little, R. (Eds.). (1997). *Relatives Raising Children: An Overview of Kinship Care.* Washington, DC: Child Welfare League of America.

Curtis, P. A., Leipold, M. & Petit, M. R. (1995). *Child Abuse and Neglect: A Look at the States: The CWLA Stat Book.* Washington, DC: Child Welfare League of America.

Davidson, B. (1997). Service Needs of Relative Caregivers: A Qualitative Analysis. *Families in Society, 78*(5), 502-510.

Drake, B., & Yamada, G. N. (1996). A structural equation model of burnout and job exit among child protective services workers. *Social Work Research, 16*, 104-129.

Dubowitz, H., Feigelman, S., Harrington, D., Starr, R., & Zuravin, S. (1994). Children in Kinship Care: How do they Fare. *Children and Youth Services Review, 16*(1/2), 85-106.

Fortune, A. E., & Reid, W. J. (1999). *Research in Social Work* (Third Edition). New York: Columbia University Press.

Genty, P. (1998). Permanency Planning in the Context of Parental Incarceration: Legal Issues and Recommendations. *Child Welfare, 77*(5), 543-559.

Gilbert, N., & Terrell, P. (1998). *Dimensions of Social Welfare Policy.* Needham, MA: Allyn & Bacon.

Gleeson, J. (1999). Kinship Care as A Child Welfare Service. In R. L. Hegar, & M. Scannapieco, (Eds.). *Kinship Foster Care: Policy, Practice, And Research.* (pp. 28-53). New York: Oxford University Press.

Hornby, H., Zeller, D., & Karraker, D. (1996). Kinship Care in America: What outcomes should policy seek. *Child Welfare, 75*(5), 397-409.

Ingram, C. (1996). Kinship Care: From Last Resort to First Choice. *Child Welfare, 75*(5), 550-566.

Jackson, S. M. (1999). Paradigm Shift: Training Staff to Provide Services to Kinship Triad. In R. L. Hegar, & M. Scannapieco, (Eds.), *Kinship Foster Care: Policy, Practice, And Research* (pp. 93-111). New York: Oxford University Press.

Mandelbaum, R. (1995). Trying to Fit Square Pegs into Round Holes: The Need for a New Funding Scheme for Kinship Caregivers. *Fordham Urban Law Journal, 22,* 907-936.

Scannapieco, M., Hegar, R., & McAlpine, C. (1997). Kinship Care and Foster Care: A Comparison of Characteristics and Outcomes. *Families in Society, 78*(5), 480-491.

Scannapieco, M., & Jackson, S. (1996). Kinship Care: The African American Response to Family Preservation, *Social Work, 41*(2), 190-196.

Takas, M., & Hegar, R. L. (1999). The Case for Kinship Adoption Laws. In R. L. Hegar, & M. Scannapieco, (Eds.), *Kinship Foster Care: Policy, Practice, And Research* (54-70). New York: Oxford University Press.

Tutty, L. M., Rothery, M. A., & Grinnell, R. M. (1996). *Qualitative Research for Social Workers*, Needham Heights, MA: Allyn and Bacon.

Ways and Means Committee Print WMCP: 105-7. (1998). *1998 Green Book.* Section 11. Child Protection, Foster Care, and Adoption Assistance. (Online). <http://www.gpo.ucop.edu/>.

Zwas, M. G. (1992). Kinship Foster Care: A Relatively Permanent Solution. *Fordham Urban Law Journal, 22,* 343-373.

A New Grandparenting:
Dialogue and Covenant Through Mentoring

Shimshon M. Neikrug, PhD

SUMMARY. The author explores the social identity of older persons and their potential for taking leadership roles in their families and communities as mentors to young persons with disability. Dealt with is the powerlessness of both these groups within society and the way in which they may be able to empower each other. It is posited that serious and active grandparenting and mentoring have the potential of filling a large gap in the continuum of meaningful and productive activities for older adults and provide highly valuable support and human resource to young persons with disabilities. *[Article copies available for a fee from The Haworth Document Delivery Service: 1-800-342-9678. E-mail address: <getinfo@haworthpressinc.com> Website: <http://www.HaworthPress.com>]*

KEYWORDS. Grandparents as mentors, leadership role of grandparents, role models for young with special needs, empowerment

The term "mentor" has become more common in usage in recent years. Mentoring is used to describe a type of formal volunteering. The model has

Shimshon M. Neikrug is Professor of Social Work, Tel-Hai College.

Address correspondence to: Shimshon M. Neikrug, PhD, Tel-Hai College, Upper Galilee, Israel 12210 (E-mail: sneikrug@netvision.net.il).

The author gratefully acknowledges and thanks David Glanz, Assistant Director at the Bar-Ilan Brookdale Program in Educational Gerontology at Bar-Ilan University, Israel, for his encouragement, insightful comments, and support on this and earlier versions of this paper.

An earlier version of this article was presented at the 5th Annual Conference on Developmental and Intellectual Disabilities, Larnaca, Cyprus, March 27-29, 1998.

[Haworth co-indexing entry note]: "A New Grandparenting: Dialogue and Covenant Through Mentoring." Neikrug, Shimshon M. Co-published simultaneously in *Journal of Gerontological Social Work* (The Haworth Press, Inc.) Vol. 33, No. 3, 2000, pp. 103-117; and: *Grandparents as Carers of Children with Disabilities: Facing the Challenges* (ed: Philip McCallion and Matthew Janicki) The Haworth Press, Inc., 2000, pp. 103-117. Single or multiple copies of this article are available for a fee from The Haworth Document Delivery Service [1-800-342-9678, 9:00 a.m. - 5:00 p.m. (EST). E-mail address: getinfo@haworthpressinc.com].

103

also been used by business and industry as a form of tutelage or sponsorship of a young worker by a more experienced worker as part of on the job training. Freedman (1993) traces the use of the term to its classical roots. In Homer, Mentor, is an old friend of Odysseus who protects and guides his only son Telmachusin in his father's absence. Later, the goddess Athena, who was associated with wisdom, takes on the guise of Mentor, to help guide the young man through his adventures.

In this paper the concern is with common problems shared by two groups: young persons with a disability and older adults. Society places constraints on the behavior of it members. Normative limits are placed on everything from dress, to speech, and to behavior. Often young persons with disabilities and older adults violate these norms by their very being in society. It was not so long ago that asylums and "homes" existed to make both young persons with disability and older adults as invisible as possible. Often it still seems as if the community would prefer to return to the 19th Century, when the old and disabled were placed out of sight and out of mind. Goffman, in his definitive work on the subject of stigma, states, "Social deviants, as defined, flaunt their refusal to accept their place and are temporarily tolerated in this gestural rebellion, providing it is restricted within the ecological boundaries of their community" (1963, p. 145). In this view, young persons with visible disability, or old people, are social deviants and, they "flaunt" their differentness by their very being. Social deviants are temporarily tolerated in their community until collective fear creates a situation where "something has to be done." Most often, in the past, the "something" means separation.

Today we know that there are other means of separation than physical separation by institutionalization. Hazan states, "The separation of the aged from society, the identification of aging with ugliness, evil, and horror, and the reluctance to engage in physical contact with the aged all indicate that aging is perceived as a dangerous area located, as it were, between life and death" (Hazan, 1994, p. 69). Society seems afraid of all social deviants. Deviant groups share the experience of rejection by their communities and can be tolerated in a "gestural" rebellion as long as their differentness remains restricted to acceptable norms. They may try and "pass" into the normative majority. The old may try to conceal their age. They use cosmetics to alter their skin and hair and attempt a "youthful" life style. This is generally approved of by society and they are given support for being so "young." The young person with a disability may also attempt to pass, hiding their disability in numerous ways. However, in truth, both groups are physically, as well as socially marked. What is more; they are socially ubiquitous. They are not, as other minorities, bounded by class and caste. They are with us all: rich/poor, Black/White, peddler/professor.

Here what we are concerned is with the powerlessness of these two groups and the ways in which they may be able to empower each other. We seek to understand the potential for older persons taking leadership roles in their families and communities as mentors ("elders of the Judeo-Christian tradition; wise men and women") to young persons with disabilities. We do not purport to present a finished set of plans for our program, or a set of empirical data. Hence its value lies not in its immediate utility, but rather as conceptual tool, opening up new possibilities in the field of inter-generational activism.

Our approach is based on an awareness of the similarity of experience shared by these stigmatized groups and the potential strengths of elders to reconstruct their old age and, at the same time, support young persons in their self-work.

The work of reconstruction is facilitated by dialogue. As Freire posited, "The pursuit of full humanity . . . cannot be carried out in isolation or individualism, but only in fellowship and solidarity . . . "(1972, p. 58). We are concerned with the potential of dialogue between senior adults, dealing with their experience of stigma, and the need of adolescent and pre-adolescent young persons with disability to develop as a mature and whole self. We call this dialogue 'grandparenting'. Grandparenting can take many forms. The form that we wish to consider in this paper is grandparenting as mentoring. We are also concerned with the potential of older persons who are not related, to become mentors and develop solidarity with young persons with disabilities. We often use the terms grandparenting and mentoring interchangeably to emphasize the fellowship that is available to all older adults through this form of caring.

THE PROBLEM WITH GRANDPARENTHOOD

When we think of senior adults, their adult children and their grandchildren, what often comes to mind is a complex interaction of expectations, demands, responsibilities, duties, and values that often result in conflict and dissatisfaction, painful scenes of confrontation or hurtful avoidance of open expression of feeling. It has been argued that the harmony between the generations depends on an elusive balance between the autonomy and dependence between senior adults, their adult children and their grandchildren (Werner, 1991). But what are the rights, duties, and responsibilities of grandparents? What happens if these are in conflict with those of parents? What is the area of autonomy and independence for grandparents? Do they continue to have responsibilities and duties to their adult children? Can there be an independent grandparent/grandchild relationship? Finding an area of *independent* action across the generations is the goal of many grandparents. Many grandparents fear that their self-esteem is endangered if they are to become subservient to their adult children in all things that pertain to their grandchildren. These seniors wish to fulfill a family role that is senior.

Gerontological research that has studied the concept of the grandparental role has been less than optimistic regarding older persons' abilities to find a meaningful role in the modern family. Clavan (1978) attempted to euphemistically describe the grandparental role as an "ideological" role; a role without rights or responsibilities. Hazan (1994) is even more explicit. He states, " . . . the concept of role (is) inappropriate as a focus for the analysis, description, and understanding . . . " of the world of the grandparent" (p. 42). He argues that the dependency and negative self-image of the elderly is highlighted by the fact that their only true reciprocal relations are with grandchildren, who by definition are also powerless.

Kornhaber is also pessimistic regarding much of contemporary grandparenting. He states, "Only a minority of grandparents in the study has a close relationship to a grandchild," a finding that could not be explained by geographical distance alone (1996, p. 37). He therefore hypothesized that there exists a new social contract that distances grandparents from grandchildren. While the social forces that separate grandparents from grandchildren may be on the wane, it still seems that grandparents often fear that involvement will be interpreted as meddling, interfering, or controlling. It even seems that the symbolic idea of "grandparent" is more important to elders than the acts of grandparenting. "They spend their time thinking and daydreaming about grandchildren and display their pictures, like trophies of their existence, whether or not they are intimately involved in the child's everyday life. . . . they fill their consciousness with a . . . nostalgic daydream. . . . Grandchildren often do the same, generating ideal images of grandparents" (Kornhaber, 1996, p. 52).

Rosow (1973) argued that the social status of being defined as a grandparent does not provide the individual with a normative social role telling him or her how to act and what was expected behavior by society. Moreover, grandparents are often disregarded in studies of the family. For the most part, when we hear the term family, we imagine a nuclear nest of parents and their immature children. This is true despite of the growing number of families with at least one grandparent and in many cases, even with great-grandparents.

Kivnick (1988) categorizes the "dimensions" of the grandparenting relationship. Among the dimensions she identifies is that of the "valued elder" with emphasis on the passing of cultural traditions the grandchildren and the establishment of "clan." Other studies (Gutmann, 1985; Neugarten and Weinstein, 1964) have also emphasized this aspect of grandparenting: older person as link to the familial and tribal past. Even a "well-rounded" senior adult with many life interests may still place great meaning upon the grandparent-child relationship as a locus for the passing of the flame between the generations, taking his/her place as the head of the clan, and being responsible for personal and familial continuity. In this dimension lies the possibility of immortality of the elder through the continuity of the family, but this dimension may take a rather passive form, requiring little more of the grandparent that simply being there.

A NEW GRANDPARENTING

As was indicated at the outset of this paper, grandparenting will be considered as a way of using the human potential of older adulthood. It seems that being a grandparent is the perfect avenue for this kind of meaningful self-expression, and that mentoring is the best vehicle for navigating that too rocky road.

Mentoring adds a new dimension to meaningful grandparenthood. Grandparents are able to hew out meaningful position in the modern family. They enter into a relationship that places the focus on the grandchild, but in which both grandparent and grandchild are equal beneficiaries. Mentoring can be a main life challenge and opportunity for the elder who is willing to use this accrued wisdom to support the growth and development of a child; especially a child with a developmental disability. Work by Kornhaber and Woodward (1981) may have been the first study to have listed mentoring with the roles of grandparenthood. Kornhaber (1996) adds to the term mentor words such as: nurturer, crony, soul mate, wizard, hero, and spiritual guide. These dimensions are sources of meaningfulness in most, if not all, grandparental relationships. Freedman (1993) deals with mentoring by persons who are not relatives that he refers to as 'the kindness of strangers.' In 1989, The National Mentoring Partnership and United Way of America convened a representative group of organizations with significant experience in running mentoring programs. They defined responsible mentoring programs as those programs, which meet the needs of both the mentored participants and the volunteer mentors. Responsible mentoring is a structured, one-to-one relationship or partnership that focuses on the needs of the mentored participant. It fosters caring and supportive relationships, encourages individuals to develop to their fullest potential, and helps an individual to develop his or her own vision for the future.

The art of mentoring involves listening to youth, creating "youth-driven" relations, building relationships over time, respecting personal boundaries, being sensitive to differences, focusing on the youth, providing support and challenge, acknowledging reciprocity, and being realistic. It also requires a re-engagement with the realities of the urban community as well as other larger social policy reforms.

The common elements of the idea of mentoring are: achievement, nurturing, and generativity. Due to the pressures on the modern family and the collapse of the traditional social structure of the neighborhood, youth are often cast adrift in a world devoid of close adult relationships. These young people are often alone and alienated; this may particularly apply to youth with developmental disabilities who are also often alone and alienated because of their differentness. Mentoring is perceived of as a way to make a difference in their lives through the creation of a significant human connection. Its advantages seem clear: mentoring seems to be a simple, direct, sympathetic, legitimate, and bounded way to help young people. It is posited that serious and active grandparenting and mentoring has the potential of filling a large gap in the continuum of meaningful and productive activities for older adults and providing highly valuable support and human resource to the young. The obvious advantages of mentoring are readily observed, but less attention has been paid to the role of the grandparent for the psychosocial development of the young person with disability. When serious and active grandparenting and mentoring takes place vis-a-vis young persons with disability, the social value of the activity is multiplied many times over.

By becoming a significant adult friend, the mentor can make a difference by supplying information and opportunities, as well as nurturing and support, to the young person–helping to prepare him or her for adulthood, by passing on coping skills and experience. Numerous and powerful forces in society combine to project a negative and hurtful image of disability. In the mentoring relationship with grandparents, a place is created where the young person with disability can find allies to assist in the development of a more whole and powerful self-image. Inclusion in the schools is important but it is not enough. A loving nuclear family is essential but not sufficient to develop to assist young persons with disability to develop an authentic identity in the face of the majority environment. Children and teenagers with disabilities need all the resources that can be mustered today to achieve a healthy development. Grandparents could become powerful allies in this struggle. Grandparents can fill a critical gap in the development of the inner life of these youth while, at the same time, meeting their own needs for a powerful and meaningful identity.

CONTEXT

The ideas presented in this paper are based on our work and the work of our colleagues, with older adults in innovative programs in Israel. Over the past decade, there has been a concerted effort to understand the contributions and needs of grandparents, and to offer support programs. In Israel and in other countries, programs have been established that offer training and education for older persons on "becoming better grandparents," and "achieving grandparent potential" (Strom and Strom, 1988, 1989, 1990, 1997).

We have drawn upon the experiences of three Israeli programs with which we have been involved. More information on the three programs may be obtained by writing to the author. The first of these is a university-based program, teaching senior adults community organizational skills and encouraging them to take positions of active leadership in their communities. Currently we enroll thirty senior adults in the program each year. In the last nine years approximately two hundred older persons have participated in this course. During the course they are exposed to the needs of children with disability, and are offered opportunities to take leadership positions in agencies that serve young persons with disability.

The second project is an Israeli version of the Family Friends Program. This program was "imported" from the U.S.A. where it is sponsored by the National Council on Aging (NCOA). With the assistance of NCOA, we initiated a program for informal volunteerism for older adults. They become "friends" of families challenged by a disability. This program was mounted in a large day program for children with a developmental disability.

The third project is another application of the Family Friends model geared to families who had been afflicted by disability through acts of violence. In Israel, these families are served by the National Institute for Social Insurance. The staff at the National Institute for Social Insurance realized that in addition to the need for formal support (emotional, as well as, financial) there is often a need for informal support for families challenged by traumatic disability. During the last four years, one hundred and twenty "friends" entered families that had indicated a desire for such intervention.

The Family Friends Programs tend to be very informal. The families and the friends are expected to be independent of bureaucracy, much as natural friends are. There is little data collection and statistical follow-up. Much of what we know is derived from interviews with the directors of these programs. From their narratives we find several shared approaches and themes:

- The programs described here are characterized by relatively low turnover as compared to other programs that encourage friendly visiting.
- The families are given information about the possibility of a "friend" being introduced to them, but they are under no pressure or expectation to agree. While there is a mechanism for either side to request a re-assignment, only 15% of placements are unsuccessful.
- When placements are successful, the tendency is for the relationship to last for years.
- The volunteers represent a fairly broad range of demographic characteristics, but the range is skewed to the young elderly, of middle-class backgrounds, and with average or better education. However, in all the

programs there are participants that differ greatly from the modal description.

- In all the programs the "volunteers" are given a far greater degree of freedom of activity than is typical of volunteer programs in Israel. The volunteers and the families become "friends" rather than representatives of the agency and their clients.
- All of the projects have a training component, lasting between a few months up to an entire year, that is geared to foster independent volunteerism.

Finally, much of our knowledge about mentoring comes from the author's own support system which continues to give him understanding, insight, and encouragement to be a mentor to his own grandson, challenged by a disability.

Each of the programs mentioned includes a formal learning component. Over the years a learning style has developed that characterizes this work. It begins with a "contract" between "teacher" and participants that they will strive together to invent a learning relationship based on solidarity unlike anything experienced in past learning situations. Courses are based on an attempt to incorporate these values in the learning process.

A basic theme of these courses is that personal experience is as valuable as the formal course content. The crux of the educational experience is the finding of the universal in the students' life experience. Their significant experiences are the "generative themes" which are the real content of the learning dialogue. Experience has an elevated place perhaps even above "book learning" in the hierarchy of truth. The awareness of the needs of older learners to improve their status, increase their self-esteem and self-efficacy, and strengthen their cultural identity has led to the development of a style of learning and an educational strategy for:

1. recognizing learners' strengths,
2. promoting their ability to develop new ideas and approaches,
3. strengthening their ability to make their own future choices,
4. assisting them to work better with others, and
5. increasing their ability to access valued resources (Kindervatter, 1979; Hughes, 1987).

We found that meaningful learning with these older adults best takes place within an experiential, dialogical consideration and study of the meaning of aging for the participants. This "study" of the personal experience of aging has also been found to be an empowering experience for the participants. As one participant said in her best college English, "This has been balm to my soul."

None of the programs described were intended to promote mentoring activities. The feedback we received from our students regarding their developing relations with their families led to an understanding that the new strengths developed in the learning situation often lead to mentoring. This led us to consider how these strengths could be intentionally directed to mentoring activities by programmatic intervention.

THE PRACTICE OF GRANDPARENTAL MENTORING

Mentoring, like so many important things in human experience, is usually observable only by its effect upon the system in which it is located. Studies show that among persons in the Ojibwa tribe, the greater amount of time a grandfather spent as carer, the better the child's grades in school and better social functioning (Williams et al., 1996). A study on grandparent-grandchild contact in China also found a positive relationship between contact and academic performance and positive personality (Fablo, 1991). Similarly, Burnette (1998) designed a group intervention for Afro American and Latino grandparents and found a resultant increase in problem solving and support seeking in grandchildren and a decrease in depressive symptoms. Kivnick (1986) found that the grandparental figure was central to the subjects' sense of ego ideal.

Although we are able to document the results of grandparental mentoring, we are often frustrated by the question, "But what is it? How is mentoring done?" The grandparent mentor in native American society has been the subject of several childrens' books and portrays the grandparent as responsible for the transmission of traditions, ceremonies and beliefs (Smith-Trafzer and Trafzer, 1988; Neihardt, 1972; Niatun, 1995).

These stories show that in traditional societies there was a role for elders, but they are unable to provide much insight into the "how" of mentoring. They do, however, point out the importance of myth and the spiritual as basic to the mentoring relationship. This is more clearly seen in Bly's book *Iron John* (1990). Bly proposes that identity is transmitted by the "old myths" passed by elder mentors to the young. He states in the preface to the book, "The images of the old stories . . . finding the Wild Man under the lake water, following the tracks of one's own wound through the forest and finding that it resembles the tracks of a god–these are meant to be taken slowly into the body. They continue to unfold, once taken in." Bly goes on to say, "The ancient societies believed that a boy becomes a man only through ritual and effort–only through the 'active intervention of older men'. It's becoming clear that manhood doesn't happen by itself; it doesn't happen because we eat Wheaties. The active intervention of the older men means that older men welcome the younger man into the ancient, mythologized, instinctive male world."

Along with the content of the myth the verbal language itself is of great importance. Kutter (1996) points to this in her discussion of helping children deal with pain. She states, "Language that conveys any degree of support, hope, love, courage, energy, or appreciation, and that promises at least some release from suffering helps children to let go of their fear and pain. . . . As you actively attend to a child's language and behavior, you teach yourself to respond to his or her message" (p. 93). Without language, the child experiences pain for which there is no meaning. In the absence of meaning, the child places the context of the experience in the magical (i.e., the pain is punishment for my breaking a taboo, it is the act of a baneful god, or the magic of an imaginary enemy.) The use of language in the mentoring process is a way of dealing with pain so that the mythical and the symbolic are able to replace the magical. The unraveling of the myth provides the clue to finding meaning in the experience. Experience, no matter how painful, is more manageable when it becomes meaningful.

The combination of mythical content and the language are often best understood in the form of dialogues. The psychotherapist Albert Kreinheder, in his discussion of his own passage through disability and disease, invents an imaginary mentor who he names Kieffer and with whom he enters dialogues. One dialogue with Kieffer is about the pain in his foot from which he finds no relief no matter what treatment he attempts.

> The imaginary Kieffer responds, "'Well, of course . . . the real issue is with the symbols . . . . What image does it raise in your mind? . . . '
>
> 'I see an old man hobbling with a cane.'
>
> 'What kind of a person is he?'
>
> 'He's very alive mentally. . . . a kind of philosopher . . . people come to him because he inspires them . . . '
>
> 'So . . . you see . . . The problem is that you have been unaware of the interesting old man. So perhaps the foot trouble is there so that you would limp . . . so that you would get a feeling of his presence, even for a time feel a bit like him yourself. His presence will probably change you quite a bit.' (1991, pp. 47-48)

Kreinherder is an older man mentoring himself. To understand the image behind the symptom, he brings a lifetime of wisdom and understanding in the form of dialogue. Through the dialogue he is able to conceptualize an inner meaning to the pain he experienced, and more importantly, he is able to actively ask the questions that are the basis of the dialogue.

Brown and his associates, in their research on empowerment of persons with disabilities found that most people with disabilities did not see themselves as making any improvement in their rehabilitation. They found clear evidence that the client's fears and concerns were not dealt with. They found that the result of interventions by staff were to play down activity and reduce the responses of clients' to the confines of the rehabilitation alone. The opportunity for developing empowerment, so necessary for the rehabilitation to succeed, is lost. They conclude, " . . . rehabilitation is not about keeping people quiet, but about enabling people to express themselves . . . " (1992, p. 3).

The mentor encourages dialogue. Mentoring is about enabling. The feedback we have received from our older participants has made it clear that there are universal experiences shared by both them and their young "client." These are the same experiences that were grist for the dialogues analyzed by the participants in the learning programs. They relate to the condition of differentness. The following are two brief dialogues presented by grandfathers of children with physical disabilities:

"Grandpa are you sad to be old."

"Do you think it's sad to be old?"

"I think so."

"Why?"

"Because old people become ugly."

"Am I ugly?"

"No, but other people . . . "

"Why is that?"

"Because old people are different. People don't like people to be different."

"Why is that?"

"Grandpa you're lucky to be old."

"Why is that?"

"Old people don't have to work and people give them their seat on the bus."

"Why is that?"

"Because people feel sorry for old people."

"Why is that?"

The dialogues deal with the response of society to differentness and they are prologue to the basic questions; why am I different? Can I handle and perhaps succeed in the challenge of my differentness? Is there positive meaning in a life as a person with differentness? The mentor is able to allow the expression of the young persons' search for meaning when he or she has dealt with the oppression of ageism and struggled to find meaning in their own lives. What is necessary is the identification and reification of these universal experiences. These are the building materials out of which positive identities are constructed.

CONCLUSION

The style of intergenerational action presented here is empowerment. The awareness of the need of both older adults and young persons with disability to improve their status, increase their self-esteem and self-efficacy, and strengthen their identity has led to suggesting mentoring as a means of using grandparenting to result in empowerment for both. In grandparent mentoring both older adult and young person with a disability "learn" empowerment through mastering issues of authority, responsibility, community, and developing a willingness to attempt to change.

We see grandparent mentoring as a still evolving form. It is a process that begins anew with each generation as older adults and young persons with disabilities strive together to invent a relationship that is not like anything experienced in the past for either. Their significant experiences are "generative themes" which are the real contents of a meaningful life dialogue and a powerful tool to deal with the alienating influences to which both older adults and young persons with disabilities are so vulnerable in our society. We have found that the empowerment resultant from understanding one's personal experience with oppression and ageism can be the basis for courageous support of young persons challenged by disability. Our challenge now is to develop programs that will harness this resource and direct it to other pressing social problems such as custodial grandparents, and problems of modern living that place young persons with disabilities at increased risk.

REFERENCES

Bass, S.A. (1987). University and community partnerships: Developing linkages for quality gerontological training and institutional expansion. *Educational Gerontology, 13*, 307-324.

Battersby, D. (1987). From andragogy to gerogogy, *Journal of Educational Gerontology, 14*, 4-10.

Bly, R. (1990). *Iron John: A book about men.* New York: Vintage Books.

Brown, R.I., Bayer, M.B., and Brown, P.M. (1992). *Empowerment and developmental handicaps: Choices and quality of life.* London: Chapman & Hall.

Claven, S. (1978). The impact of social class and social trends on the role of grandparents, *Family Coordinator, 27,* 351-58.

Cross, W.E. Jr. (1991). *Shades of black: Diversity in African-American identity.* Philadelphia, PA: Temple University Press.

Freedman, M. (1993). *The kindness of strangers: Adult mentors, urban youth, and the new voluntarism.* San Francisco, CA: Jossey-Bass Publishers.

Freire, P. (1972). *Pedagogy of the oppressed.* New York: Penguin Books.

Glanz, D. and Mayer, E. (1977). American Jewish religiosity: A new perspective–Modern orthodoxy and the Jewish counterculture. *Forum of the Jewish people, 35,* 117-131.

Glanz, D. and Neikrug, S. (1994). Making life meaningful. *Aging International, 21,* 23-26.

Goffman, I. (1963). *Stigma: Notes on the management of spoiled identity.* Englewood Cliffs, NJ: Prentice-Hall.

Greenspan, S.I. (1997). *The growth of the mind and the endangered origins of intelligence.* Reading, PA: Addison-Wesley.

Gutmann, D. (1985). Deculturation and the American grandparent. In V.L. Bengston and J.F. Robertson (Eds.), *Grandparenthood.* Beverly Hills: Sage.

Hazan, H. (1994). *Old age: Constructions and deconstructions.* Cambridge University Press.

Herzog, A.R. (1989). Age differences in productive activity. *Journal of Gerontology, 44,* s129-s138.

Jendrek, M.P. (1993). *Grandparents who parent their grandchildren: Findings and policy implications.* Miami University, Oxford, OH.

Kivnick, H.Q. (1988). Grandparenthood, life review, and psychosocial development. *Journal of Gerontological Social Work, 12,* 66-81.

Kornhaber, A. (1996). *Contemporary Grandparenting.* Thousand Oaks, CA: Sage Publications.

Kornhaber, A. and Woodward, K.L. (1981). *Grandparents/grandchildren: The vital connection.* Garden City, NY: Doubleday.

Kreinheder, A. (1991). *Body and soul: The other side of illness.* Toronto: Inner City Books.

Krutilla, J.O. and Benson, D.E. (1990). *The Reflected-Self Identity of Learning Disabled Adolescents: Perceptions of "I Am" Using Symbolic Interaction.* Paper presented at the International Conference of the Learning Disabilities Association (Anaheim, CA, February 21-24).

Kuttner, L. (1996). *A child in pain: How to help, what to do.* NY: Hartley & Marks.

Lowey, L. and O'Conner, D. (1986). *Why Education in the Later Years.* New York: Lexington Books.

Manheimer, R.J. and Snodgrass, D. (1993). New Roles and Norms for Older Adults. *Educational Gerontology, 19,* 585-595.

Medding, P.Y., Tobin, G.A., Barack Fishman, S. and Rimor, M. (1992). Jewish identity in conversionary and mixed marriages. *American Jewish Yearbook 1992*. American Jewish Committee and Jewish Publication Society, New York, NY.

Minkler, M. and Roe, K.M. (1993). *Grandmothers as caregivers: Raising children of the crack cocaine epidemic*, Newbury Park, CA: Sage Publications.

Moody, H.R. (1990). Education and the life cycle: A Philosophy of aging. In R.H. Sherron and D.B. Lumsden (Eds.) Introduction to educational gerontology. New York: Hemisphere Co.

Morris, R. and Bass, S.A. (1986). The Elderly As Surplus People: Is There a Role for Higher Education, *The Gerontologist, 26*(1),12-18.

Mullen, F. (1995). *A tangled web: Public benefits, grandparents, and grandchildren*. Washington, DC: AARP.

Neikrug, S. (1998). Releasing senior potential: Lessons from our learners. *Aging International, 24*, 287-298.

Neihardt, J.G. (1972). *Black Elk Speaks. Being the Life Story of a Holy Man of the Oglala Sioux*. Lincoln, NE: University of Nebraska Press.

Neugarten, B.L. and Weinstein, K. (1964). The changing American grandparent. *Journal of Marriage and the Family, 26*, 199-204.

Pilley, C. (1990). *Adult Education, Community Development and Older People Releasing their Potential*. London: Cassell Educational Ltd.

Priestley, M. (1995). Commonality and difference in the movement: An "association of blind Asians" in Leeds. *Disability-and-Society, 10*(2), 157-169.

Rein, M. and Salzman, H. (1995). Social integration, participation, and exchange in five industrial countries. in S.A. Bass (Ed.). *Older and active: How Americans over 55 are contributing to society.* (pp. 238-262). New Haven: Yale U. Press.

Rosow, I. (1973). The social context of the aging self. *Gerontologist, 13*(1): 82-87.

Rothenberg, N. (1997). *Jews in Israel and the United States: Diverging identities*. Paper presented at the International Workshop on Jewish Survival: The Identification Problem at the end of the 20th Century," at the Sociological Institute for Community Studies, Bar-Ilan University, Ramat Gan, Israel, March.

Schachter-Shalomi, Z. and Miller, R.S. (1997). *From age-ing to sage-ing*. New York: Time-Warner.

Schoenfeld, S. (1997). *On theory and methods in the study of Jewish identity*. Paper presented at the International workshop on Jewish survival: The Identification problem at the end of the 20th Century, at the Sociological Institute for Community Studies, Bar-Ilan University, Ramat Gan, Israel.

Schweid, E. (1994). Changing Jewish identities in the new Europe and the consequences for Israel in Webber, J. (Ed.), *Jewish identities in the new Europe*. London: The Littman Library of Jewish Civilization.

Shuldiner, D. (1992). The Older Student of the Humanities: The Seeker and the Source. In T.R. Cole, D.D. Van Tessel, & R. Kastenbaum (Ed.). *Handbook of the Humanities and Aging.* (pp. 441-457). NY: Springer.

Smith-Trafzer, L.A. and Trafzer, C.E. (1988). *Creation of a California Tribe: Grandfather's Maidu Indian Tales*. Newcastle, CA: Sierra Oaks Publishing Co.

Streicker, J. (1997). *Why family matters: Community, class, and culture in the making of Jewish identities*. Working paper from the Brandeis University Institute for Community and Religion, San Francisco, CA.

Strom, R. and Strom, S. (1988). Intergenerational learning and curriculum development. *Educational Gerontology, 14*, 165-81.

Strom, R. and Strom, S. (1989). Grandparents and learning. *International Journal of Aging and Human Development, 29*, 163-69.

Strom, R. and Strom, S. (1990). Raising expectations for Grandparents: A three generational study. *International Journal of Aging and Human Development, 31*, 161-67.

Strom, R. and Strom, S. (1997). Building a theory of grandparent development. *International Journal of Aging and Human Development, 45*, 255-86.

Tager, M. (1984). Looking into the whirlwind: A psychohistorical study of the Black Panthers. *Psychohistory-Review, 12*(2-3): 61-70.

Thomas, C.W. (1987). Pride and purpose as antidotes to Black homicidal violence. *Journal of the National Medical Association, 9*(2): 155-160.

Thompson, W.J.A. and Cusack, S.A. (1991). *Flying High: A Guide to Shared Leadership in Retirement.* Burnaby, B.C. Canada: Simon Fraser University.

Webber, J. (1994). Modern Jewish identities in Webber, J. (Ed.), *Jewish identities in the new Europe.* London: The Littman Library of Jewish Civilization.

Werner, E.E. (1991). Grandparent-grandchild relationships among US ethnic groups. In P.K. Smith (ed.) *The psychology of grandparenthood: An international perspective.* London: Routledge.

Williams, E. et al. (1996). Grandfather involvement in childrearing and the school performance of Ojibwa children. *Merrill-Palmer Quarterly, 42*, 578-95.

Index

Abandonment, parental, 38
Adoption, by kin caregivers, 19,47,
    73-74,87,91,98-99
Adoption Assistance and Child
    Welfare Act, 87
Adoption Assistance and Safe
    Families Act, 87,91
African-American children, percentage
    in kinship care, 18
African-American grandmother
    caregivers
    for grandchildren with special
      needs, 4-5
    historical background of, 37
    negative impact of caregiving on, 3
African-American grandparent
    caregivers, 2,111
    demographics of, 37
    hypertension in, 27
    negative impact of caregiving on,
      3-4
Age
    of children in kinship care, 19,73
    of grandparent caregivers, 4,18,25,
      45,69,72,92
AIDS (acquired immunodeficiency
    syndrome), parental
    effect on children's health, 40
    as reason for grandparent
      caregiving, 25-26,38-39,89
Aid to Families with Dependent
    Children, 88
Alaska, kin guardianship program in, 91
Alcohol abuse
    by grandparent caregivers, 3
    by parents
      as cause of children's disability,
        89
      as reason for grandparent
        caregiving, 39

Anemia, in grandparent caregivers,
    27-28
Anxiety, in grandparent caregivers, 3-4
Arthritis, in grandparent caregivers,
    27-28
Asthma, in grandparent caregivers,
    27-28
Athena, 104
Attention deficit hyperactivity disorder,
    in children in kinship care,
      4-5,24,30-31, 47-48,73-74
    diagnostic criteria for, 23
    parental substance abuse-related, 40
Autism, of children in kinship care,
    47-48,73
    parental factors in, 40

Baltimore, Maryland, kinship foster
    care in, 87-88
Behavioral disorders
    of children in kinship care, 4-5,20,
      47-49
    of foster-care children, 21
Behavior management training, for
    kinship foster caregivers,
      96-97
Brookdale Foundation, 60
Budgeting assistance, for grandparent
    caregivers, 76,79

California, kin guardianship program
    in, 91
Case management, 45,65,68,77,88-89
Caucasian children, percentage in
    kinship care, 18
Center for Epidemiological Studies-
    Depression Scale (CES-D),
      3,43

TO ORDER: CALL: 1-800-429-6784 / FAX: 1-800-895-0582 (Outside US/Canada: + 607-771-0012) / E-MAIL: getinfo@haworthpressinc.com

☐ **YES**, please send me **Women as They Age, Second Edition**

___ in hard at $69.95 ISBN: 0-7890-1125-5. (Outside US/Canada/Mexico: $84.00)

___ in soft at $24.95 ISBN: 0-7890-1126-3. (Outside US/Canada/Mexico: $30.00)

Signature _____

☐ **BILL ME LATER** ($5 service charge will be added).
(Not available for individuals outside US/Canada/Mexico. Service charge is
waived for/jobbers/wholesalers/booksellers.)

☐ Check here if billing address is different from shipping address and attach purchase
order and billing address information.

☐ **PAYMENT ENCLOSED $** _____
(Payment must be in US or Canadian dollars by check or money order drawn on a US or Canadian bank.)

☐ **PLEASE BILL MY CREDIT CARD:**

☐ AmEx ☐ Diners Club ☐ Discover ☐ Eurocard ☐ JCB ☐ Master Card ☐ Visa

Account Number _____

Expiration Date _____

Signature _____

THE HAWORTH PRESS, INC., 10 Alice Street, Binghamton, NY 13904-1580 USA

NAME _____

INSTITUTION _____

ADDRESS _____

CITY _____

STATE _____ ZIP _____

COUNTRY _____

COUNTY (NY residents only) _____

E-MAIL _____

May we use your e-mail address for confirmations and other types of information?
( ) Yes ( ) No. We appreciate receiving your e-mail address and fax number. Haworth would like
to e-mail or fax special discount offers to you, as a preferred customer. We will never **share, rent, or
exchange** your e-mail address or fax number. We regard such actions as an invasion of your privacy.

☐ **YES**, please send me **Women as They Age, Second Edition** (ISBN: 0-7890-1126-3)
to consider on a 60-day **no risk** examination basis. I understand that I will receive an
invoice payable within 60 days, or that **if I decide to adopt the book, my invoice will
be cancelled.** I understand that I will be billed at the lowest price. (Offer available only
to teaching faculty in US, Canada, and Mexico.)

Signature _____

Course Title(s) _____

Current Text(s) _____

Enrollment _____

Semester _____ Decision Date _____

Office Tel _____ Hours _____

(06) (17) 05/00   BIC00

FAX